On the Machine

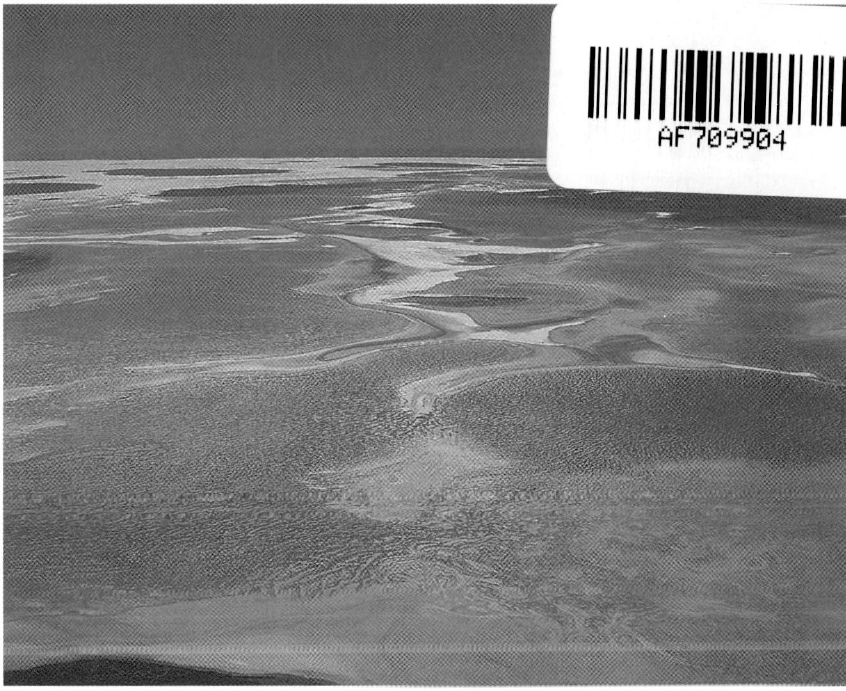

Aboriginal stories about kidney troubles

Compiled and edited by
Jeannie Devitt and Anthony McMasters

jukurrpa books

First published in 1998 by
IAD Press
PO Box 2531
Alice Springs
NT
0871

National Library of Australia Cataloguing-in-Publication data:
On the machine: Aboriginal stories about kidney troubles.

ISBN 1 86465 003 6.

1. Chronic renal failure — Patients — Australia, Central.
2. Aborigines, Australian — Diseases — Australia, Central.
I. Devitt, Jeannie. Living on medicine. II. Devitt, Jeannie. III. McMasters, Anthony. IV. Title: Living on medicine.

362.19661400899915

Design: Louise Wellington
Map: Brenda Thornley
Printed by Sands Print Group in Australia

Cover photograph of Lake Mackay by Peter Latz

foreword: a personal message

I didn't know my kidneys were failing—I didn't know until last year—November last year. At the start I was told to come [to] Alice Springs Hospital but I didn't know this thing—they have to put it in the arm; they call it a 'fistula'. They said, 'We going to put a fistula in you because your kidneys are not working.' From there I [felt] a bit worried because my kidney—it's going to ruin my body. And so they put the fistula in and they said, 'You going to start to go to dialysis and be a renal patient.'

At first—day one—they did it in hospital, before I went down to Flynn Drive [Community Centre]. That was after Christmas I started up my dialysis [there]. I was doing this [in] January, February, March—three months in a row for the dialysis—[then] I had to go to Darwin. In Darwin I stayed for a couple of weeks.

They said, 'No, you got to stop here for six months.'

'Who said so?'

'That mob in Alice Springs.'

'No, I'm not stopping here for that long! I'm going back! I was told by them Alice Springs [people] I'd be up here for two weeks only.'

[I returned to Alice Springs.] Then...I was all right. I was going Tuesday, Thursday and Saturday, that's all my days—the days I have to go in for my dialysis. Unless, if I'm going away somewhere for meetings or family visit, I have to come in an extra day...That's what the nurses told me...'If you miss the dialysis you gotta be sick.'

A lot of people have been doing that; they've been doing that because they haven't got understanding. [Some] other people think it's going to make it better if [they go] away just with no reason, without telling the nurses or doctor. That's why some people just pass away. The nurses don't realise why the renal patients die; [it's] because people worry for their family, their country and to be there with their family close by. That's why they get worried—worry and stress—they get [that] a lot, and then they get sick because of thinking you know, [like if] other family passes away in the community. See, I lost three family [members] in a row. I don't worry [about not attending funerals] because I'm a dialysis patient, I don't worry, but people—some people—*do* worry, they stress out, you know by thinking a lot of things—family things.

People can only go home for a short visit, maybe one or two days, maybe three days; before doing that they have to go to dialysis and get extra thing done to the body, then they can go out; thinking [about] not to have any more fluids while they're out in the communities. That's the thing—people drink a lot, lot of water, tea, cool drinks, some even drink grog...I've seen this happen, and I wonder why the nurses or the doctors don't encourage people; [really] they don't. [Some encouragement,] something that they can be happy...

I'm involved in community things like Council and I help the CAT [Centre for Appropriate Technology in Alice Springs] and I help local government [bodies]; I do little bit of interpreting between the community and the government agencies. So I'm busy. When there's a meeting coming up, I have to organise myself with dialysis before I go out [bush]. If I do that, the nurses will be happy because I'm doing the right thing; some people don't do the right thing, they just take off. But I had to think [about] my dialysis *before* I think [about] other things...For me, something is working...my feeling is better because I'm having to go back to communities a lot, that makes me happy. For other people, I don't think they do that. [Maybe] some do.

I know there's one old man [on dialysis] who's been happy all the time, he's a renal patient, he's happy all the time. But sometimes when he's sick, he [doesn't] talk to anybody. Especially when there's a problem, they don't tell; people don't tell because they're too sick to say, they are too sick to talk about what is causing them to be sick...

I was trying to help—I mean to talk to the nurses—the people in charge of the renal clinic and, you know, everybody is too busy doing their job. I haven't seen anything for renal patients, any good things like what I think [would be] encouraging people to be happy. The staff works and the renal patients just go there and get on the machine for four hours or four and half hours sometimes, and that's the end of it until the next two days. There's no time for finding out [anything]—nurses or someone in charge of the renal clinic should be asking people: 'Are you happy, are you sick, or worrying?' It's very disappointing I think myself...because these staff are not talking to these renal patients. I always wonder why they're doing this...

The doctors said they gonna put me on the list for a kidney transplant. It might come in a year's time, or it might be couple of years. It's a two years waiting period but it might happen before. There are people who were here for *ten* years—they were asking the same question—just the personal questions, talking to one nurse. [The nurse] said, 'Oh, you better wait till next time, when kidneys become available.'

I don't think [the staff really] understand because if patients and the nurses talk to each other [then] I feel happy, they feel happy. I don't know what their feelings are like...I don't know what [the staff] think, and they don't know what I think. My feelings are different from their feelings. I feel very strange when I'm in town...But if they [want to do] something for sick people—renal patients—they should be listening and communicating to people, talking—make people happy, make people feel better. And people should have a dialysis bus—renal patients should have a bus to go out to communities and have a visit. And that way the patients are happy, family are happy in the community, everybody's happy...

The first time when people come in—the first warning they get is: 'Now you're on dialysis, if you go away for a week or four days...you get sick and you die.'[1] That's the warning, that's the first message we get from the nurses...Sometimes family comes into town to visit—that's not enough. You know if there's business on—there's business happening in communities—people got to be there to practise. See, I'm still making up my plan to get out to Kintore on Christmas holidays but they can only allow me for three days.

It's really the kidneys problem. If that wouldn't be a problem I could be [at Kintore] all the time...The [local] health services talked about putting a dialysis thing on the community—they all support it—even the health staff, the community, everybody, even the doctor. All they're waiting [for is] to see if they get the money from ATSIC Regional Council—or from somewhere. They put in for the funding in the health budget, they put in for a new health clinic—and with that they can have a space for a dialysis machine.

I now want to make a statement about renal patients. I want to give a message to anyone who listens to this and support us with the idea: People on dialysis need to get back out there to their communities for cultural reasons, to be there with their family, to be there with the other relations and make themselves happy. All we renal patients should have this chance to go out and have a visit. We need to know [we can do] that. We don't have any hope for us, for ourselves. We [need] to have a dialysis machine out in a community, that way people can be happy in their country and with their family. That's the message I wanted to give—that's my personal message. I don't know what the other people think. If nobody [else] is going to say something about [renal patients'] lives, they [themselves] should say. But I am talking for myself and also for those other renal patients. This is the message I'm giving.

Smithy Zimran Tjampitjinpa
Alice Springs
December 1997

1 In later conversation this was likened to being spoken to 'like a dog'.

Contents

Acknowledgments

We would especially like to thank the Aboriginal renal patients—both in Central Australia and those in Western Australia—who, along with their families, gave their time to help us better understand their situation. Though they remain anonymous here, their words will speak to all who read them.

We also repeat our thanks more generally to the large group of individuals—mentioned by name in *Living on Medicine*—for their assistance with the research, the community visits and the final reports. Here it is particularly important to recall those who helped with language and interpreting: the Institute for Aboriginal Development's Language Centre; David Nash, Jenny Green, Gavan Breen and Myfany Turpin of the Institute for Aboriginal Development's Dictionary Project, and John and Katie Heffernan of Yirara College.

Pam Lofts provided the artwork used during the course of the research; at short notice she revised and drew additional illustrations for this publication.

The research and associated training program was conducted under a grant to Central Australian Aboriginal Congress from the National Health and Medical Research Council. Additional literature research and revisions preparatory to publication were possible through a grant from the Australian Institute for Aboriginal and Torres Strait Islander Studies. Finally, the Commonwealth Department of Health and Family Services, Office for Aboriginal and Torres Strait Islander Health Services made this publication possible.

Introduction

Alice Springs is a small town; its population is only around 30 000. From the time local renal care facilities were established in 1987, those directly involved in patient care have been aware of the difficulties facing Aboriginal renal patients. As the numbers of Aboriginal renal patients have rapidly escalated so too has community anxiety, leading to—among other things—calls for haemodialysis facilities in remote communities and regional centres. In response, Central Australian Aboriginal Congress, a community-controlled Aboriginal Health Service based in Alice Springs, and the Central Australian unit of the Menzies School of Health Research jointly proposed, as a preliminary step, an investigation of the situation of Aboriginal renal patients. They successfully sought funding from the National Health and Medical Research Council in 1993; the research began in mid-1994 and the resultant report, *Living on Medicine*, was finally completed in late 1996.

The researchers were concerned that the report, written in what many local Aboriginal people refer to as 'hard' or 'big' English, would be virtually impenetrable to the majority of patients. This volume, *On the Machine,* is a companion to the main report. It has been compiled in an effort to bring at least some of the material directly to the patients, their families and communities. It is an edited selection from the interviews which formed the basis of the research, including commentary from Aboriginal patients, family members, Aboriginal kidney donors and knowledgeable community members. This volume also includes a series of illustrations that were initially used to focus discussion and elicit comment during interviews. They have been revised and rearranged into a series of illustrative stories for *On the Machine*. We hope *On the Machine* is a catalyst for discussion among renal patients and their families about the major issues confronting them, as well as a useful resource for the broader Aboriginal community.

home communities of all patients

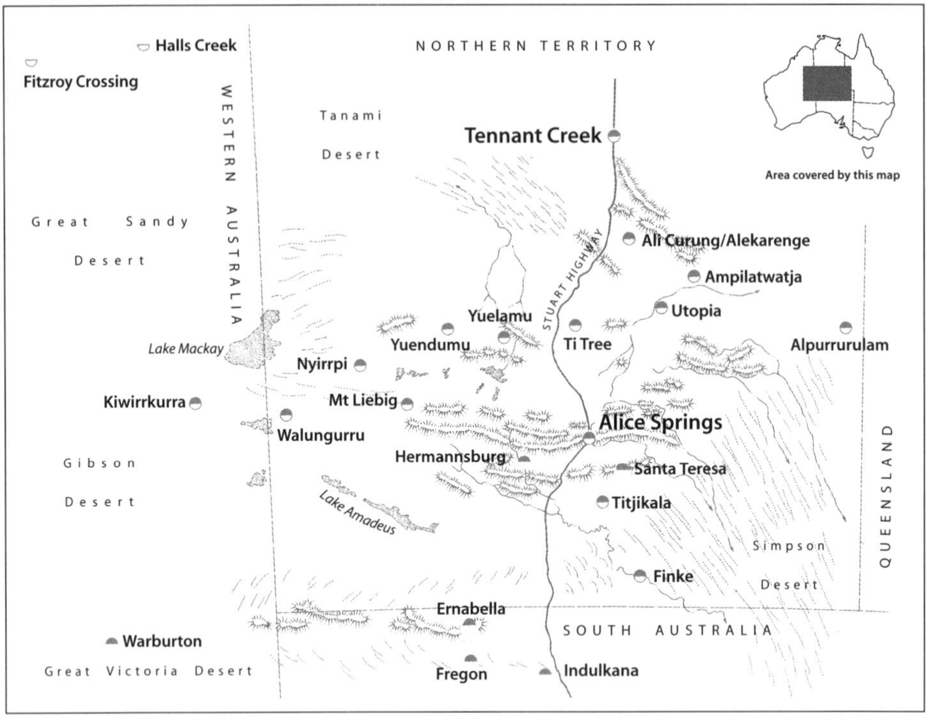

Patients' community of origin

Community visited by researchers

List of special words

the 'bag'	a soft plastic bag used for CAPD. A set comprises one empty bag into which the fluid from the peritoneal cavity is drained, and one full bag of a special fluid that is used to fill the peritoneal cavity. This fluid is the dialysing agent
bogey	bath, shower, wash, swim
CAPD	continuous ambulatory peritoneal dialysis: a form of dialysis that is not dependent on complex technology and can be carried out by patients in their own homes; often referred to by patients as 'the bag'
Congress	refers to either of two Aboriginal community-controlled medical services in Central Australia: Central Australian Aboriginal Congress in Alice Springs, and Anyinginyi Congress Aboriginal Corporation in Tennant Creek
finish-up business	mourning rituals, also referred to as 'sorry business'
Kardiya	European, Whitefella, used particularly in the Western Desert communities
the machine	the haemo-dialysis machines
marlu	kangaroo (Warlpiri language)
mukaki	black plum, *Santalum lanceolatum* (Warlpiri language)
ngangkari, ngangkayi	Aboriginal healer, 'doctor', 'cleverman' or 'medicine man' (in Warlpiri and Arandic languages; there are equivalent terms in other Central Australian languages)
PD	peritoneal dialysis
peritoneal	refers to the peritoneal (abdominal) cavity; the dialysis fluid is drained into, then out of, this space around the organs in the abdomen
pirlirrpa	spirit, soul, life-force (Warlpiri language); and (for some Warlpiri speakers) mind, feelings, disposition, attitude
rations	in this context, a term for the kinds of food that Central Australian Aboriginal people received from White people during their earliest contacts: a limited range of foods including tea, sugar, flour, jam, golden syrup etc.
strong (bag)	the dialysing fluid in the CAPD bags comes in various strengths, and sets of bags are differently numbered accordingly. Patients refer to bags by their numbers
Yapa	Aboriginal person (used in the Western Desert area)
yarda	sorcery sticks (Warlpiri language)

they had no kidney problems in the early days

Lena Apwerl,[1] a community leader and a senior health worker of 15 years' experience, considers whether or not earlier generations had kidney disease.

They had no kidney problems in the early days, [their kidneys were] completely free of disease. People just died from things like old age—maybe from being without meat and getting weak. [Then] their foods were bush potato, bush bananas and banana leaves, sugarbag [wild honey] and honeyants...that's what they always lived on.

[People] with diseased kidneys probably have blood problems—and they get it from sugar—that damages them. They *will* keep on drinking soft drinks—that's the problem. Earlier people had none of these—they were really healthy, they had no problems [like today]. They lived on just sugarbag and on kangaroo and goanna.

But, if they *did* get sick, others would sing over them and use healing massages—like the *ngangkari*—casting off the sickness; singing and massaging away the sickness, just continuously massaging them...making them cool, cooling them down with their singing.

Those people weren't sick, they were always healthy, they didn't have [these kinds of] diseases; they never knew about this kind of sickness—this kidney disease.

Well, cool drinks—the sugar—that's what causes kidney problems, makes them stop working. The old people used to eat brown sugar—I'm talking about earlier, when the first White people came—well, that [kind of sugar] was okay...At first they used to just watch those White people. They say they used to go around looking for them [to watch them] and they became more familiar with White people, [they saw how] they ate brown sugar and bread. [White people were living] out here in these bush places then—over that way...Well they only had rations—they used to give out wheat—not that white flour, no, it was brown flour. They were good, those foods they used to live on.

(Translated from Anmatyerr by J. Devitt)

1 All Aboriginal people named have been identified with permission.

Now they get sick for good

A group of four women, who are all senior community figures actively involved in community development issues, gathered at the Yuendumu Women's Centre to talk about whether earlier generations suffered from kidney disease. They explain the meaning of pirlirrpa *(spirit) and why it's important for health.*

Uni: *Yirdipirrki* means 'kidney'. Well, a long time ago, [Aboriginal people] used to be healthy—when they lived before White people came. When they used to get sick...with bad kidneys, well the *ngangkari* would fix them up.

They used to say, 'Oow, why am I in pain? My kidney is hurting.'

'Maybe you woke up too suddenly from your sleep. Maybe you got a fright from the dog, or someone might have shouted loudly while you were asleep.'

'Yes, that's why I got sick. Can you get someone to come with a *ngangkari* so he can make me better?'

That's what people used to say, long ago. Before White people's food, [Aboriginal] people used to fix themselves with the *ngangkari*. They used to fix their kidneys and they'd get better, but today people are getting sick with kidney problems and they're on medication—and on machines. A long time ago they used to be really healthy because they had plenty of healthy food—bushtucker—that's how they made themselves healthy—even the little kids were made better by the *ngangkari*. People had their *ngangkari* to look after them and fix them.

They used to go out hunting; they'd ask each other, 'Hey, are you feeling better today?'

The sick one would reply, 'Yeah, you made me better. I'm feeling a lot better today.'

'Yeah, all right, that's good news,' the *ngangkari* used to say.

The sick person would feel better straight away, thanks to the *ngangkari*. The *ngangkari* used to say [of] that sick person, 'Maybe they were getting bad inside when they were getting full-up—blood-wise.' Because today people get sick from eating different kinds of food that belong to non-Aboriginal people, that's why they get sick. And now they have doctors and sisters to look after them.

We're telling stories, we're talking to this lady who came here from Alice Springs. We're talking about sick people everywhere who have kidney problems. *Pirlirrpa* [spirit], that's what we call 'kidney'.

They used to get sick. When they were fast asleep, dogs would bark and [people] would jump awake quickly [i.e. were startled]. But when[ever] their *pirlirrpa* was no good, the *ngangkari* would make them better straight away, and the next day they would be walking around happily.

Ruth: [They had] really strong healing powers.

Uni: In the early days, before the White people, people had their own *ngangkari*, but these days, *Kardiya* time, there's only a few left.

Ruth: Yes.

Uni: Now [Aboriginal people] get sick for good.

When they went hunting, they would dig for bush potatoes and kill goannas and the men used to go for kangaroo...they used to get sugarbag. They used to go out hunting all the time, that's how they used to make themselves strong. They used to be healthy but now things are getting worse through *Kardiya* people's food—because we eat lots of sweet food. When we ate honeyants and sugarbag we never got sick, though—people got strong from eating them.

We used to have honeyants, sugarbag, goanna and black berries. And they used to get lots of seeds, called *yukarrija, wurlumpuru* and *yika*...and mulga seeds. Our fathers used to give us lots of seeds to grind to make damper. We would grind the seeds with our mother and grandmother, and today we still have that law. We still have bushtucker today—we didn't forget them. We get sick from eating White people's food.

We might get sick, that's why we always eat bushtucker. Doctors and sisters know about bushtucker.

Long ago when people used to find it hard to [find] bushtucker, the old people would sing the land for more. The land would become green, and there would be plenty of bush potatoes. People were really healthy and their blood was strong, but today our blood is no good from all the bad food.

Ruth: We used to have strong blood.

Uni: They had healthy kidneys, they fixed each other with *ngangkari*—

Ruth: —[with] *ngangkari* and women's ceremony and songs...They sang each other.

Uni: They had a special *marlu* song to heal people when they were sick and the *ngangkari* would ask them, 'Are you feeling better now?'

The sick person would answer, 'Yes, I'm feeling much better now. I'm feeling strong now.'

Even when their spirit goes away from their body the *ngangkari* fixes them. They used to put the spirit back [in]to the sick person's body. The sick person would [then] eat lots of bushtucker.

Ruth: [When] you have no spirit, you're empty, maybe there's something wrong with you.

Uni: [Your spirit is] gone—

Ruth: —yeah, you have no spirit, it's gone. The *ngangkari* would tell the sick person, 'You have no spirit.'

Uni: There used to be one clever *ngangkari* who did this—

Ruth: —the *ngangkari* would say to the sick person, 'Maybe I'll try to get your spirit back to your body.'

Uni: Lots of people had *ngangkari* [i.e. there were many healers].

Ruth: In the early days, *ngangkari* were clever—they used to know where the spirits were...The *ngangkari* used to rub the spirit. He would put the spirits back into their body, and the sick person would feel strong after that.

Uni: [*demonstrating*] Like this, Nangala [interviewer]...

Ruth: The sick person would say, 'It's true, he fixed me.'

Uni: [The *ngangkari* rubbed them] with dry fat mixed with water.

Ruth: 'Yeah, your spirit was [away from you] there,' [the healer would say].

Uni: 'Your spirit was a long way away,' the *ngangkari* used to tell him [patient] and he'd tell the sick man's family that he was better.

When there was trouble, [Aboriginal people] used to get sick through jealousy, you know—

Ruth: sometimes—

Uni: —yeah, sometimes. People used to be enemies—a long time ago—

Ruth: —sometimes people damage other people's kidneys through Aboriginal business—

Uni: —and they can clear away their sickness [like that] too.

Ruth: Before, they used to hide each other's spirits [i.e. cause a person's spirit to disappear from them]—

Uni: sulkily [out of resentment]—

Ruth: —or maybe the husband used to do this. Husbands used to make their wives sick because of [their wife's attraction to] another man—

Uni: —and they used to blame him. In the early days a young girl would be promised to a man. She would live with her parents before getting married. If the girl didn't want to marry her promised husband, the man would get upset and do something to the girl's family. He would make them sick.

Nowadays, people are forgetting about promised husbands because we're living the White people's way.

These day young girls don't like getting married to their promised husbands, they go the other way—their own way...These days babies are born when sisters and doctors are around. [Before] if a man and a woman ran away—being lovers not promised to each other—they would get speared, or sometimes they would be made sick from *yarda*. It was like that all the time. The mother and father of the girl would only like the girl's promised husband, that's *Yapa* [Aboriginal] way.

People used to say, in the early days, when a girl wasn't interested in marrying her promised husband, they'd say, 'Why did she turn away from him? She's breaking the law.' But the man would let her go anyway. The man would go to another place where his family was, and his family would ask him, 'What happened? Where's your wife?' His family used to feel sorry for him, and they would make that girl sick with *yarda*.

Today we have two laws: *Yapa* law and *Kardiya* law. Today when we get sick we have medicine. Before when they got sick *ngangkari* made them better. They would bring the sick person to the *ngangkari* and he could make them better straight away. They used to sing them to get better and strong. That's how they lived long ago.

When people used to get sick with *pirlirrpa* and when they had kidney problems, the *ngangkari* would fix them straight away. Long ago they had their own *ngangkari.* Whenever a person got sick a *ngangkari* would fix that person straight away, but today we have White people's medicine and also they have special tablets these days. That's all I had to say.

(Translated from Warlpiri by the Institute for Aboriginal Development)

they never leave me by myself

N.A., a dialysis patient, and some of her family members talk about N.A.'s situation. Present were N.A.'s sister, P., her daughter, R., her daughter-in-law, some grandchildren and her son. The interview was conducted on the lawn outside the hostel where N.A. lived in Alice Springs.

N.A.: Listen to me: I'm feeling quite well now. I'm staying in the one place now, here at [the] hostel. Every day I go to the machine, they come and pick me up. I go there and I find out whether I'm improving. When I get home from the machine, I feel better—even my stomach feels better. I want my family to listen to me, to know that I'm feeling better.

At the machine they put a drip in my arm; that cleans out the rubbish inside my body. The drip is really good, it makes me feel better. It's not a bad thing. The machine cleans our stomach. I go there every day. It's really good because the machine cleans my blood. I'm much better than I was before.

They take the drip off and give me injections. Sometimes they give me medicine and I take it happily.

I was sick at [community Y.], I didn't get sick anywhere else, just at [community Y.]. Then I came to Alice Springs, and I don't go anywhere...

P.: It's my turn to talk now. I'm helping N.A., who got sick at [community Y.]. The *ngangkari* didn't make her better, she got better here in town. She used to be really healthy before, she worked at all kinds of jobs—back when she only had one daughter...

When she was at [community N.] they didn't make her better, nor at [community Y.]. It was only later in town that they made her better.

Even in Hidden Valley [Alice Springs town camp] she didn't get better. I want to tell my family—she can't go [home], she has to stay here or she might get sick again. Don't worry, we are taking really good care of her, the kids and me, Jangala, Nangala, Japangardi, Napangardi and we two Napurrurlas. We're all looking after her.

We've been talking about how she was sick before. It wasn't a *ngangkari* that made her better, it was White people who saved her. They clean her blood and body and she feels stronger after that. Good food like apple juice and lemon juice are making her stronger. People get better by eating good foods. She can't go out to [community Y.] yet, not until they say it's okay—maybe later. There's plenty of time for her to go to [community Y.] when she gets better.

N.A.: I used to be as healthy as a White person until *yarda* made me sick. My body got all swollen, my arms and legs swelled up. I was really very sick then but I'm a bit better now. The sisters help make me better, looking after me every day, but you know it was only one thing— the kidney machine—that really made me better. It wasn't a person who made me better—it was that machine. I don't skip going to the machine.

I stay here so that I can go on the machine. I have lots of tablets too that I get every Tuesday. I always take those tablets three times a day: at supper time, at breakfast time and at lunch time. I don't throw them away—those medicines make me better. They often give me injections in the stomach if I'm sick—not when I'm okay, though. If I start feeling bad the sisters give me those injections.

All my family look after me—all my kids—they never leave me by myself here, they're around all the time—the whole lot of them.

P.: Yeah, our family looks after us. They're not drinkers. We have fun. We send our kids to school, and they listen to us. We get visits from family from all over the place...We have lots of family coming into town as well as family here—they see us and make sure we're all right.

We moved away from Hidden Valley, to get away from drunks—they kept hassling us. It's better here, there's no drunks, so we're staying here. There's plenty of food here, all the family come and see us and there's lots of kids. We're happy here.

[N.A.'s] stomach used to be all swollen up before—but she's got better here; she was much worse before but now she's much better, she's more lively.

R.: It's my turn to talk now. I drink, but I still look after my mother. I might go a long way away—as long as my kids look after her—but I always come back because I worry about her.

P.: When she gets sick, we ring up the ambulance straight away. Like that time her legs got swollen up. We thought she had a boil. When we rang the dialysis unit they told us that she'd gone into hospital for an operation. Later on [we] went to visit her in hospital. So when she gets sick or swollen up we ring the ambulance straight away now.

But she's getting more like her old self now—lively. She's content because she's got all her family here. Whenever she's sick, we get the ambulance. Those medicines make her better—at the moment she's active and well. She's happy now she's got her family here, she's lively.

(Translated from Warlpiri by the Institute for Aboriginal Development)

then something will happen...

What follows is part of a conversation between two men, J.I. and A.A., from the Western Desert area. Both men have been on haemo-dialysis for a period of years. Present also were J.I.'s wife and John Heffernan (a non-Aboriginal interpreter), who asked the questions. The men debate the causes of kidney disease.

What do the family say?...Do they think [this sickness is] from sorcery? What do they think?

J.I.: What are you saying—the kidney becomes non-functional from being sorcerised?

Do they speak like that?

J.I.: Do kidneys become non-functional like this from sorcery?

A.A.: No, no.

Do they think like that?

A.A.: No.

J.I.: What do you mean? When a family member dies? [I.e. after a death people frequently blame the death on sorcery. This is probably the thought behind this question.]
I have heard some people say about someone who is in hospital, 'Why is he sick like this?' And another will say, 'He is sick because he has been sorcerised.' That is what they say.

J.I.: No, it's not like that they say—but it might be from sorcery. If [the person's kidney] were sorcerised, [the healers] would see the object in it, cut me open and get it out. They couldn't see anything in my kidney, even with the X-ray. They couldn't find anything.

A.A.: They can see kidneys and they can operate and take them out, just like they take them out of bullocks.

J.I.: Then [the medical personnel] say it has become blocked up by itself.

A.A.: —from sugar, from drinking alcohol.

A long time ago when the now-dead people were in the bush, did kidneys become bad then?

A.A.: No...they were okay. Maybe it's from sugar?

J.I.: Don't talk about that any more.

A.A.: They [were] well because they ate kangaroo and drank its blood.

J.I.: Don't say that [because we don't really know]. People became sick and it could have been from kidney problems—we don't know about these things—

A.A.: —there were no doctors.

J.I.: —because there [?was] no medicine for it, and no machines. Maybe some people died in the bush because their kidneys were not working. People used to be boned in the Aboriginal way by powerful men. That's why we used to have sick people who would then die.

A.A.: They used to get very thin and die. But now doctors can see the problem.

J.I.: Doctors can see the problem. It's good they can...

This man [referring to A.A.] *has said that he's become sick from drinking alcohol and from too much sugar. What do you think? Why have you become sick?*

J.I.: No, I only drink beer. I have drunk beer twice.

A.A.: He doesn't drink now.

J.I.: Beer is all right to drink.

Why do you think you have become sick?

J.I.: I've been following the man-making law ceremonies [initiation ceremonies] all over the place.

A.A.: No, it's not law. He's asking you, is it from sugar or drink that you've become sick? You should say things like that...

J.I.: No—it's not those things...I got sunstruck [in the summer time when a lot of the man-making ceremonies are held]. It's maybe because of that that my kidneys are not functioning. Because the sun has been overheating me for a long time. Maybe it is also from my drinking a lot of sugar in my tea. It might be that, I don't know. It might be the hot sun that's made me bad.

A.A.: It's from sugar and drink.

J.I.: Maybe my kidneys have stopped functioning because of drink. Is that true?

Yes, perhaps—what do you think?

J.I.: Do kidneys stop functioning because of alcohol?

What do you think? And what are your family saying: is this sickness from a sorcerising object?

A.A.: It's from sugar.

J.I.: No, [a certain] family caused it because they made a lot of trouble for me...If I'm dying from a sorcerising object, might be something else has happened to me.

A.A.: It's sugar, it's sugar.

J.I.: If a person keeps going around the place with man-making ceremonies, he keeps going and going to them, then something will happen...As a result of that finally my kidney has become non-functioning. That's why it's happened, because I've travelled everywhere.

When you became sick did you go to see [Aboriginal] doctor men?

J.I.: [Yes.] They were working on me. They were trying to heal me. They would work on me and they said something—what was it? They said, 'Maybe someone has sorcerised you from a far-off place.' They weren't speaking the truth. No person has sorcerised me.

Tjungarrayi [*speaking to interviewer*]! Will I tell you [how I came to be on the renal program] now without wasting any time? About going over there and finishing the ceremony at Kintore—no at Kiwirrkura—[then] we went over there to Punmu...Then after that the business mob came and they met together at Kiwirrkura. Then we left there and went on and we camped on the road that night. What is the name of the water place that we stayed at?...yes, [K.]. We all slept there at the bore. We slept there, got up and then we met with the Docker River mob before heading to Warakurna [Giles]; then others joined with us [there]. We ate food there and slept until morning, then we went on our way...

After that we went to Warburton. Then others came together with us there. Then we moved on and others joined us, then again others joined us. Then we went to [another place]. We finished [the ceremonies] there. Then we went on [travelling] again. [Several days and nights later]...after I had finished with the ceremonies there, the [Aboriginal] doctor men there tried continually to make me well but they couldn't.

A.A.: It was there that he became very sick.

J.I.: I was very weak there.

A.A.: They took him to hospital.

J.I.: Then I went to Kalgoorlie. I lay there in the hospital at Kalgoorlie. A doctor there worked on me at night. There at the hospital a woman said, 'This is only a small hospital here; you should go to a big hospital in Perth.' She said, 'If you stay here in this hospital you might die, you should go to Perth.' The doctors there said, 'Do you want to go to Perth?' I said, 'Yes I'll go.' Then the Whitefella said, 'Yes, then he'll go to Perth.' There in Perth I stayed at the hospital for three weeks...

Then to Alice Springs?

J.I.: Then they said to me, 'Don't come back here, you go there'—Alice Springs. There the sisters looked after me. That's a big city there in Perth—one can easily be lost there. It's not like this town here, there's lots and lots of people and houses and cars. I [have] stayed here in Alice Springs a long time. Then the Whitefella came and said to me, 'You're going to Adelaide.' Then I went there. It was here [indicating his arm] that they operated on me when I was down there...so that I could be put on a machine. They cut me here so I could go on the machine. The Whitefella's very clever. Those Whitefella doctors know about these things. I stayed there for two weeks...

[to J.I.'s wife*] Did you know about this man going to Perth?*

J.I.: She was staying at Kiwirrkura.

A.A.: She didn't know what to think.

J.I.: No, she cried there for me because they wrongly thought that I was dead...They rang from Perth about me to here—to Alice Springs Hospital. Then from the hospital they rang Kintore. Then from Kintore they rang to Kiwirrkura. They said that I had died. Therefore, [the family] heard that message and cried for me—yes, it was wrong. Then after that I came and stayed here [Alice Springs].

(Translated from Pintupi by Ken Hansen and John Heffernan)

they put a name on that bloke

A dialysis patient, L.D., describes how people can be made ill in an Aboriginal way. He says that this is what happened to him.

In [community Y.], I been get sick there—Aboriginal way, you know, I didn't know what happened. *Yapa* way, they just draw people [*drawing in the sand with his finger as he spoke*]...that's the way people get sick—they do that Aboriginal way, that's how I got sick. Other people got one kidney [transplant and then] they get bigger [but] after I been get one—still skinny; some people gettin' bigger, I'm still the same, 'cause man...did the wrong thing [to me] at [community Y.]...

When did that happen to you?
Long time ago. We can still talk about this at [community Y.]...people think they can kill me, reckon I'm [?myall, i.e. ignorant, easily tricked]. People do that. They draw [on] trees—[we] can't see them, we from long way, [then] people [like us] get skinny, really skinny. Like at [community L.], people do that, it's bad—really bad.

Why do people do that?
I don't know why. They get from cigarette you know [?butts], [burn] them; they can cut your hair with scissors—[then] they put a name on that [particular] bloke. Anybody can do that—older people you know...

I'm thinking only one way—I was good, working, you know, [then I] been get sick from that man now. I want to talk about [it] in a meeting—find out why I been get sick. That [other dialysis patient], they put something on his boot new boot—that's why he been get sick, he can't walk—[he's] sick [crippled] on two legs...Same time me and him been get sick—he got a lot of family...

Some doctor can't tellem what sort of sickness I got, [but] I'm worrying what sort of sickness. When I go to the hospital, he should tell me, [but] he can't tell me—he's worrying about for kidney, liver—but other thing [I'm worried about] he can't tell me. But I'm all right. After every four weeks I can come back. I can only trust one doctor...he's only going to give me medicine. I was thinking a lot. People die when they do that [sorcery]. They can do that [at these two communities they] draw on tree. That's really true, I can tell you.

a lot of worrying for the family

This is a summary of commentaries from three women related to one another—two sisters (F.R. and T.N.) and a cousin—recorded at various times throughout the project. The two sisters, F.R. and T.N., are 'the last two sisters' of their family. Their older sister (P.B.), a renal patient, has already passed away and their brothers and sisters all have diabetes.

F.R.'s story

[My sister had returned from Darwin and] she was real healthy, and was working in the school...She was okay then. All her kids were at school, her [husband] was [working] at housing association, our other sister was with us too. She [P.B.] ended up at [community E.]—that's where her kidney failed. [About two or three years prior to the interviews.]

[Then my sister P.B.] was in Adelaide. I rang her up, she just wanted to get through it...We only knew about [her sickness] when she went down for a fistula, I had to help her. I told her to go for her little boy's sake; we was both crying. I told her just go for her little son's sake...Then [she] lived in Alice Springs [on dialysis]. [She would go to community T. to visit] and we had to put her on the bus—just for a day she came up—we'd put her back [on the bus] straight away to go back on the machine. Just now and then she was going to [community E.]. [One time] she was all swollen up. I saw doctors pressing on her heart [trying to revive her]—[My other sister] was crying. They had to get me and [her] to talk to the doctor—they told us she'd had a heart attack and the doctor said they had to give her a big needle for a plane trip to Alice Springs.

They did that and she got to Alice Springs. But when we got to the ICU [intensive care unit] she was all loaded up with drips and things—we seen her with everything on it. We thought she'd wake up like before—but she didn't. She stayed there in ICU and [my sister] stayed there with her...one week later [I] heard the news [she'd passed away]. The doctor from Congress came and told me to come to the phone. So they took me to the phone to hear from [my other sister]—I couldn't believe my ears.

T.N.'s story

About 1980, when I had my last son, then I moved to [community T.]—that's when I started feeling myself sick...I was a teaching assistant for nine years [and when I started training], one year in 1992; I couldn't keep going. I was feeling no good in 1992 but I did the training. Then I finished work for four months, then started in the office. That's when my eye problem started, I couldn't see from one eye and I went to Adelaide. That's where they found [a kidney problem]—my blood pressure was all the time high. They checked up my kidney, had an X-Ray. When they told me that I'd have to look after myself I thought, 'Don't tell me I'm going to end up on machine like my sister [did].' She used to run away—it was a lot of worrying for the family...I tried a little bit—to look after myself—but it was too hard—[I used to eat] cordial, fried meat, not sugar just saccharine, chocolate—used to go to the shop and get hot chips and, you know, those potato [crisps].

My sister [F.R.]—she was drinking. When I went to hospital, she gave it up; even my brother he was drinking, he went back bush [i.e. gave up drinking], he's still there...Sometimes I get sick of it, but I push myself—I never missed one [treatment session] yet. I'm 36.

Later, on a field trip, the interviewers visited community A. where they met a relation of T.N.'s. She herself was also a diabetic. After talking about her situation she asked about transplants—how they're arranged and what happens. She wanted to know how she could be placed on the waiting list 'now'.

She was scared really

A woman describes her older sister's experience of becoming a dialysis patient.

Then my sister was taken into that dialysis unit and they put her on a machine. She was really really sick and ill and weak, and then my brother rang from Congress—from here—to talk to her [in Adelaide] and they put her on the phone and she was crying because she was in big shock to see herself hooked up on the machine. She was crying and really going mad and he was trying to encourage her to hang on there—from way up here—just by talking through the phone and it was getting a bit too much. We were all getting worried and—*really* sickly worried here—then we were running around to look for money.

[So] they sent me down there. I met up with my sister in the ward. She was crying and saying things, you know [like], 'I'm not going to live any more—do this, do that for me,' and I didn't take much notice because I think she'd gone a bit crazy, too, in her mind, saying silly things she didn't mean to—she was scared really, and I could understand that—and I was listening to her.

She didn't want to get on the machine—she thought she went for an operation, just to put the fistula in her arm and that was it, and they was going to put her on the machine back in Alice. But they had to put her on the machine there...[for] about a month.

I was there with her and I did everything—most of the things for her—because the nurses and doctors couldn't get through to her. So I was there doing things for her, like making her have a shower and go down to the heart machine, and get her on the heart machine, taking her in a wheelchair, taking her to Flinders Medical on a taxi, 'cause her eyes were going blind. I had to do most of the things with her—*for* her—because she wouldn't let the doctors or nurses do it for her.

...and I kept asking her, 'Why are you doing this?'

She said, 'Well, they said I was coming here just to get fistula in my arm, now they are keeping me here, I'm not stopping in this hospital.'

You know, she thought that they were just going to put fistula and send her back to Alice Springs. She was panicking in her, you know, she was going all panicky, and sort of blaming this—blaming that person. She was even telling *me* to get out of the ward, too, a few times. She was sick, I know that. I still stayed by her side and saying positive things. She said, 'I'm not staying here another week.'

I said, 'You have to stay one more week because I gotta take you over to Flinders to get your eyes [done].' You know they have to laser beam or whatever with it—because she was going blind. I said to her, 'You're only going to make things really worse if you're going to make yourself blind, we don't want a blind person to lead around, you know, the kids want you to see them!'

She was crying, 'Oh my kids, my kids.' I said, 'There you are! You're worrying about the kids, and they'll be worrying about you.' So that morning we got up real early—she was up before me, woke me up. 'Come on, let's go down to Flinders.' But it was really hard, and a few times at night I had to cry for her in the ward. We were a long way from home.

But after, we seen a few more patients coming in, couple of them might have been 16 or 17 year old. I just about cried, they were boys from the Pitjantjatjara side. I said, 'Look at these—only young kids!' It's really hard. Most people are saying in the communities, 'What's causing all these things?' They want to know, so they could try and stop their family getting this illness.

When we were sitting in that [dialysis room] and she's hooked up on the machine, I felt really uneasy, you know, and I kept looking—glancing around the room—looking at those other—I wasn't sort of relaxed. All the others were relaxed but me and her, we were sort of tense—felt out of place because they were other strange people in the room.

My big sister, she was like a mother to us when my mother passed away, you know, she brought us up on her own—all of us—my sisters and brothers and all our children. The kids are still missing her, you know, the little ones. Even the older ones, the ones that have grown up and they've got their own children and they keep asking for her and there's a lot of strain on the family here in [community T.]...

You sort of drive yourself to go

The following is an older man's account of starting haemo-dialysis in Alice Springs.

[W]hen I first got the machine put on me, I didn't know what to expect. The needles went into my arm—one [each] for the two tubes—when I got it and I laid back and the machine started up, and started pumping the blood around.

Then the nurse told me, 'You might feel a bit funny, you might feel dizziness, or you might feel aches and pains through your body, let us know straight away.'

'Right I'll do that.'

So I'm laying down there and I sang out to one of the nurses, I said, 'I feel a bit funny on the legs and arms.'

...She turned around and raced over.

I said, 'I feel hot as anything, feel sweaty and muggy,' and [I] threw the blanket off, 'Could I have a fan?'

So they brought me a fan and they put the oxygen on. Then I turned around and had a look, the blood pressure dropped, you see. So they had to put my leg up on the chair, tilted my leg up and my body down, to get my blood flow going again.

So that's the effect it had on me the first day and I thought, 'My God, *three* times a week!' And it got me thinking. After the nurses turned around and took my blood pressure, and the fan, and they put a damp cloth on my head and cooled me down, I came good again—I felt good again so they lowered the leg again and my blood pressure was back to normal.

That was the first day, very first day. I was very crook at that time. This went on for about three weeks...[although] I wasn't as bad as the first time. Next time I got on the machine I just felt crook—weak, in other words. The first time I felt like vomiting [and] all that when I was on the machine but after that—when I went through the next day—I was all right...

But I felt weak all the way, till they got me adjusted to the machine and [decided] how they should take the fluid out of my body. I think the thing was they did take it off a bit too quick the first few days, then they gradually worked it out on a slower basis. From there on I was pretty good...[Now it's] not a problem although once or twice I might get that fainting feeling, but that's because the fluid's being moved out of my body little bit quick—I know what the problem is now.

At first it was very hard to take. After that you sort of settle down and get used to it and by doing that you say to yourself that, 'Well, look, I got to go because I'm due to go to the dialysis today.' You sort of drive yourself to go...you don't want to miss any time that you're due to go there because you only make it bad for yourself.

So you wouldn't think about missing a session?

Oh, no! Once you miss a day you feel very crook, you know, and it's so much to catch up on.

Only that machine keeps us up

Three women (W.S., O.S. and T.N.) who are from the same area talk about their situation as renal patients. The interview was conducted sitting outside one of the women's houses. They talk about being on the dialysis machine.

W.S.: That [dialysis] machine make us sleep and headache and make us really tired—and I got cramp all the time from that machine...in the leg—yeah, both of them—cramp all the time. You know, you come home and have a sleep again, have a big rest and wake up about 6 o'clock [p.m.]. And the next day when I wake up in the morning I feel good. I walk around, water my garden at the back—I got pumpkin and potato growing. Yeah, I was all right this morning walking around.

O.S.: Same again [for me], I always get no good after that machine.

[*The following is translated from Warumungu:*]
When we get up after sleeping in the machine we feel dizzy. We get cramps too, in the legs and toes. Once we're back home we don't even feel like cooking a meal, we just have to lie down. After we've had a rest we can get up and cook some food, and then have another lie down. The machine makes us feel no good. After a good night's sleep, we feel fine the next day. It's just that machine that makes us feel no good.

When we go to the machine, they put a needle in our arm to clean our blood. They take out the dirty blood and put in clean blood. Then we go back home and feel weak again. We lie down, then when we feel better we get up and cook a meal.

T.N.: When I'm in the machine I'm all right, in the machine—just lay down there, watch TV, for three and half hours. The only thing I feel bad [is] when I come out—out of the machine. They take them needle—when they start take the needle off now, I start to get headache, dizzy, just sit for a little while, wait for myself to settle down.

What about those needles?

T.N.: That needle, sometimes it's painful—especially that local.

What about cramp?

T.N.: Yeah, sometime I cramp—especially on my leg down there, right foot—we shout too, for help, when we have that pain, it's very painful.

And they give you something?

T.N.: Yeah, sometime they give us hot towel, wrap us with hot towel, and the sister massage, you know.

And that helps?

T.N.: Yeah, I like the hot towel, when they put hot towel. Yeah, that's all I think.

And the next day?

T.N.: The next day I'm all right. And when I go home I feel like falling down. Sometime my husband's there to help me, take me to the room—yeah. Sometimes I end up with a weak voice, now—can hardly talk. Yeah, and then next day I'm all right now.

And what about if you miss out that treatment?

T.N.: If I missed out, well I get really sick. And I never missed out any—I'm there nearly every day.

W.S.: Person gotta die when you miss out. Lot of people did that, yeah...We can't miss that machine, we gotta go every three days. We go [community T.] for a weekend—go and visit family and get bus on Sunday coming back. Monday morning we go to machine. We go Monday, Wednesday and Friday...

O.S.: [*translated from Warumungu*] If we miss out on going to the machine, we'll get sick, and even die. So when we go back to [community T.] we're anxious about being away from the machine. We come back really quickly. It's the only thing keeping us alive. Even *ngangkayi* can't help people with bad kidneys. Only the machine can make them better, like a *ngangkayi*—he cleans us up and makes us feel better. So that's why we don't want to go too far from here. I left my home in the bush to come down here to live. But I like it here, because I don't have to worry...I'm not so sick of the machine that I'll leave Alice Springs. We're happy here, it's our home now. It's just that that machine makes us feel no good. The main thing we hate, it's the pain we feel when they put that needle in. That's all...

W.S.: I was going to [wait] for a White person's kidney but I'm getting no good from that machine, he make me dizzy and cramp all the time—when we go to machine—cramp properly! I get up and I still have that machine in my arm [i.e. attached to dialysis machine] and I got to tell them sister to make me stand up and they hold me. That heavy cramp always come to me, I got that cramp this year now. I used to have before, but [now] I started again.

They can give you something for cramp?

W.S.: They don't give us something to drink, tablet or them—something they call 'salty water'—they *say* that and [then] they forget about it.

Do you ask them again?

W.S.: No—I just walk away—they weigh me and [I] walk away—like I [did] on Monday...

T.N.: ...there's another two more there [on the machine] in our group. Not two—one—no, two in my group—afternoon—we got two [more]. They should do something about [those who've been there longer]. Some of us got problems, family can't give us [a kidney]. We got wait a long time for that list, you know—you know when we go for check-up—what they callem?—

I don't know.

T.N.: Chest and all that for you—like eyes and if we got—you know—transplant something.

I don't know. Maybe they check you up to see how you're going. Maybe they check up for transplant at the same time.

T.N.: Yeah, could be. [The dialysis unit] is getting full up—sometime there's not enough machines—some machines they broke now. I'm having reaction to that machine. You know, when I'm in that machine I have all these funny feeling, dizziness and short of breath—and them tickly thing everywhere, you know—

W.S.: —must be allergic—

T.N.: —yeah, allergic for that machine. That's why they always put two bag of them—what you call it—must be saline—they put that one flushing through first, cleanem before I go there. Twice they do it.

W.S.: I do [get] that—scratch myself everywhere.

T.N.: And I have problem with this one—look, [my] hand got swollen; they put that needle wrong way—they put the needle right near that artery here, and that [?blew] that artery and it was bleeding a lot in there. This hand got swollen quickly, I could see that hand growing—it happened last Wednesday.

W.S.: And they put ice [then].

T.N.: They put ice on top of it.

W.S.: [*showing her arm*] I still got this swollen up from Adelaide Hospital

You went to Adelaide, eh, not long ago?

W.S.: Two times I went there. First I went [because] this operation [?fistula] couldn't get better; second time I had operation in the neck here. That blood got blocked in here [arm] and they cut it through there and let that blood go—only it's get blocked.

O.S.: [*translated from Warumungu*] Yes. I'm telling the story about why we [all] go to the machine. This is a better way to explain it [i.e. in my own language]. They send me back to Alice Springs [from my community], or even sending someone else down here, they gather us up and send us down. We can't get better if we stay home. We might die without the machine. Only that machine keeps us up. That's why we're telling this story. Listen to us talking onto this tape...Listen to us talking, we've got something important to say to you!

Just to donate a kidney

A renal patient's family describe their dilemma when they were asked by a relation on dialysis to donate a kidney.

S.: Someone told [the patient] to ask one of her families to give kidney, but only problem is that [her] brothers and sisters can't give her kidney because they all diabetes—and plus niece and nephews—they drink—but us, we don't drink. And we know it is hard for people to live without no kidney.

A.: Sometimes we have problems—say if someone*[does* donate] a kidney to maybe afamily, and sometimes we think back that we might get to sick...and we don't know how to cope with one kidney. Plus, if we've never had a kidney transplant or probably had problems with our kidney, we wouldn't know what to do with them [patient relatives] unles someone come and explain to us how it is and how hard it is to get through operations and kidney transplants. Most of the time [she] gets upset, she sort of—like force us to do things—we sometimes find it real hard you know, because it's real [scary]...

And she sometimes growls at us and say[s], 'If youse don't hurry up [and donate a kidney], you know if something happened to me, don't bother about crying!' or something like that. She gets real upset—most of the time. But she's just saying, 'Probably [only] at the last minute youse'll be looking for kidney transplant.'

She's been saying this and that—and sometimes hurts our feeling which we don't answer her sometimes. We don't answer her questions—what she asks us [about donating a kidney]...she came around here about a couple of months ago, saying that she isn't very sick to stay on the kidney machine.

She said she's too sick?

S.: Yeah, she reckon one of them doctor told her that she is a bit too sick to stay on the machine, she need a kidney [transplant] for her—that's what she told us.

A.: And she said that—I don't know if the kidney specialist or probably the nurse—said that if she stays there a bit longer, the kidney machine mightn't do good for her, it's best if she get a kidney transplant from someone. Even if it's not a family, as long as there is someone there to help, and 'cause that's what she told us. We wasn't there when they spoke to her, we was here. She came from Alice Springs to here to tell us.

Did you have a talk to that kidney specialist yourselves?

A.: No, we never met with the kidney specialist yet.

S.: I would like to meet someone like kidney specialist, someone that talking to [her], because maybe she don't understand what they are talking. It's best for someone to come down here to [community T.]—

or inviting us down to Alice Springs—so that if someone talk to her about kidneys, she got someone always—like one of [us]—with her, so that we can explain, or even our dad, so that we can understand what they talking to her. Sometimes she can't listen too. She reckons she can only listen a little bit sometimes—she's a bit deaf, she can only listen little bit. If you talk to her she [can't hear]. It's better off when we get close up to her and talk—or even touch her.

A.: Best if someone is touching her—sometimes even if someone talk to her—or probably shout at her—she doesn't hear very well.

S.: So it's best for us, we need someone to come down or inviting us telling us about that machine—what it is doing too, and we want someone to talk to us telling us why and what they do—and what they gonna do about her, and what's going on with her. We need to know all those things...[She] thinks she is waiting a long time for kidney, that's why when she comes back home she get upset [with] her families.

When did she start talking to you about transplant?

S.: A couple of weeks ago she came back and she was asking if family wanted to give her kidneys.

She didn't start talking about it straight away, when she went on the machine?

A.: No. She spoke to the kidney specialist in Alice Springs and she came down and asked us for the kidney donation—just to donate a kidney and she told us that she was going to Adelaide to get it done...We asked her, 'How long will it take?' Well, she hasn't been spoken to [by] this kidney specialist yet—but if he comes back he probably will tell us what's going to happen to her.

She told you she was going to Adelaide?

A.: That [is] if she's already got a kidney donation from someone else—even though if it's from not us family but from someone else—but [it] doesn't matter which way she wants to get it, but as long as someone [i.e. the donor] is already dead.

You think it's fine for her to get a kidney from a strange person?

A.: That doesn't matter, even though if it's not family—as long as someone is already dead—just to save life. Most Aboriginal people now, they have sorrows nearly every year, more than European people does, and Aboriginal people—the young and old are dying.

What about my life?

I.Y. donated a kidney to a female relation who subsequently passed away. He talks about the experience and makes a tape-recorded statement in his own language to be played to other families considering kidney donation. The interview was conducted at I.Y.'s house.

I went down to Adelaide and [also] had a lot of tests here in Alice Springs Hospital—the dialysis place where they tested my blood and everything—everything was all matched up. But I got to say this: it's not a very good thing to donate kidney.

[Y]our life will be ruined—it's no good for young people because it's a very dangerous thing. [W]hen I done this I prayed first. Now I'm sorry what I done, you know, because she's not alive any more—she took one of my body—one of my kidneys to the grave.

And I like to say this: good luck to the other people who is getting transplant for kidneys and I'm very happy what they doing, but do not donate any because it is very dangerous.

So you think it is better for people to get a kidney from a person who is already dead?
Yes I do; especially from people who had car accident, and people that not walking any more—people that's ready to go in the graveyard—that's good, you know, 'cause it won't hurt them any more 'cause they got no sense of feelings...

[First of all] I thought it [the idea of donating] was no good. But I just said I can't lettem suffer too much, you know—'cause her father grew me up—he grew me up from a kid. That's why I couldn't turn her down 'cause he was a special man to me and she was very special to me too. [She] asked me...I done it for her 'cause [of] what [her] father done for me. That's how it worked...

Well [now] I do get cramp and everything, that's why I got to walk every time to town...when you trying to sleep at night time. I['m] just saying that's very dangerous, you got to walk around night time too, because when you cramp you can't move—and that's true story.

Did you know anything about kidney disease before you donated your kidney?
No, I didn't. That's another thing I didn't know about...I didn't know anything about kidney disease. I think they must have warned [me] down in [Adelaide's Queen Elizabeth Hospital] and Dr [B.] at Congress here, 'What you doing is very dangerous,' and my [Aboriginal] mate said the same to me too.

I said I was trying to be careful but they all said it's not a [good] thing to do. All the families said this to me, 'You be careful because you might catch disease.'...Yeah, I have to be very careful now, if I don't get this disease. If my wound come open— well that's it. I can't do nothing. [Y]ou can work in the office—lightly job, but you can't do that pick and shovel job either.

When those doctors talked to you about donating your kidney did they point out...the kind of problems you might have yourself, did they tell you that, and what did you think?

Well, they said that to me. I thought twice—but it was too late...Well they [had] paid everything for me, I couldn't refuse and...I said to her [the recipient], 'I can't do it.' That was in Alice Springs here. So I had second thoughts and I said, 'No.'

What did she say?
'Well, let's go to the doctor and see if I got disease or something in my kidneys.' And the renal doctor told her, 'One side of kidneys got disease in it, it might [infect] your body, you know.'

He said to her, 'Let's go for a big test in Adelaide.'

So we both went for a test—in the right side of the kidneys. It was really bad kidneys she had—it's very infected kidney. Well, really I didn't want to do this business, 'cause I wasn't warned—no-one told me about it until I went to Congress one day. [But] I said, 'Well, what this old man done for me, I just got to do what she want me to do for her, you know.'

So what happened is: Congress picked me up—I went in the afternoon...to the airport, my ticket was all ready to go to Queen Elizabeth Hospital. And there was no turning back.

You didn't feel like saying, 'No, I've changed my mind.'? You didn't want to say that?
I did say that, but it was too late 'cause what they said to me, 'What we paying your airfares up and down for?' So I said, 'Oh well, I'm here now, might as well get it over and done with.' That's what I said...

Well, this donating business—donating a kidney—I didn't know nothing about this, till doctors came around and told me, 'It's all ready, ready to go,' that my kidney was already passed through the machines. But when you go and do these tests, I'm just saying to youse: Be careful, 'cause these tests not very funny [i.e. it's very serious], they can kill you—and the stuff you go through is not very funny...

Some family do force people but they never forced me.

No? That was your own choice?
Well, it was really the doctors' choice. They was going to pull the machine off her, but the machine was only just going for one day, she had...only about 24 hours to live. By the time I got down there she would have been dead. But we both went into the operating theatre on the 25th of October—the 10th [month] 1993. She was dead by the time I got there but when they got the kidney into her, she came back to life again and now—she made it for 1994, but she died...And I just see lotta people go and get check-up too, you know, because it very dangerous thing, you know—specially overweight people. Doctors even told me this too. They put me on a seven-week diet—yeah, they did [*laughs*].

And did that do some good?
It did—I couldn't eat! They give you this special stuff, put it in your food and that stuff makes you weak, and your body gets weaker and weaker and weaker, just to get that weight down—and they can operate on you...

Well, I reckon it's not right to get a kidney from family—from your mother, father or daughter or your son. From a dead person it's all right, 'specially when they have a car accident. Don't matter if it's a stranger, don't matter who it is, long [as] it's here to save your life—like [that woman]—she had a kidney transplanted, eh? She got it from a bloke, from Adelaide. She died now, poor thing, and I know a lot of people in Adelaide, Queen Elizabeth Hospital, from Alice Springs, they reckon they don't want any other people's kidney.

That's what they say?
Yeah, that's what they say to me.

They want family kidney?
Yes, they want family kidney but the doctor always say, 'We can't give family kidney all the time to youse, because don't matter if it's your son, your aunty, your mother all this.' The doctors always say, 'You want to be careful, they might have something wrong with their [kidney],' like that. Well, a lot of people drink a lot of alcohol in this town, lot of grog, you know, and you know it might infect them, infect them other mob too, because [of] what the grog does to people's...body...But if it's an emergency they can get it from their family straight away. But some people—I know they're frightened.

To get it from strangers?
[*laughs*] From their family too—yes.

Oh yeah, you heard them talk about that?
Yes, I heard them, I heard them all the time, don't you worry about that!

And what did they say?
Well they say, 'What about my body, and what about my life—and I got kids to look after, and what if I go wrong something [i.e. get ill]?' That's what I heard lotta people saying that, to their mothers or fathers too sometime, you know, and I heard lotta Europeans say the same too—'What about my life?'

I want to say this in language:

Well, all you mob, [I'm telling] you, [think] very carefully—don't just rush in [and give up] a kidney. You should realise it's dangerous—really dangerous for you. It's no small thing, not something to be casual about. I know—I've had the operation myself.

I spent six months in the Queen Elizabeth Hospital—six months! I nearly died. I'm getting around okay now but I'm telling you mob, 'Don't even *think* about giving up a kidney to someone else!' Think very carefully; talk it over with the doctors at Congress first...

'Cause I know all about this business, I been through it—that's what I'm telling you mob on this tape now, be careful what you mob do. Please ask your doctors because it can be very dangerous. 'Cause you don't know what you going through, you don't know what your family gonna end up with...

(Translated from Western Arrernte by the Institute for Aboriginal Development)

I'll have the bag—more better

The researchers travelled to the Kimberleys and met C.X. She had been managing her own (peritoneal) dialysis at home for about six months. C.X. invited the local Aboriginal medical service nurse, L., to join us. After talking, C.X. showed us her treatment room and storage area.

Yeah, I was down in that place [Perth] too and I was watching them machines, you know...

They asked me, and I said, 'I'll have the bag—more better.'

And the doctor said, 'Yeah, you might as well have the bag—more better than the machine.'

...It was good too! [*laughs*].

You didn't like the machine?
No. [*laughing*] Beautiful machines, eh? But I don't know how to work them.

Yeah, well, that's right. They might have given you some training though.
No! [*laughs*]

So you're happy with this bag?
I'm happy, yeah—it's good...

When they did the training for this bag was it hard for you to understand it—or easy?
No. Easy. They showed me and they sit with me and watched me, you know; they told me how to do it first—and then I was trying my best and all—and I catch it and then they were sitting and watching me—the sisters—you know. And I'm right now. They said, 'Okay, you can go home then.'

I stayed there eight months! Just to learn and training in this bag, you know—they kept me down there for a good while you know...They didn't want to send me home early; if I don't know how to do that bag—I might get sick up here and [then] go back again...

Would you like to learn the machine?
[*laughing*] No...I like the bag, more easy...

[She describes her return home.]

Yeah, this [house] was ready for me when I was down Perth, you know. So when I came back I stayed down [at a local hostel] for four or five weeks and then I came up here.

And that's okay here? No worries?
No worries—[the nurse] come and see me every time. [*laughs*]

*[*addressing L.:*] How often do you have to come over?*
[*L.:*] Once a month to do a stocktake and count up—count up everything and then phone it through to Sydney.

*[*addressing C.X.:*] Where do you keep all those bags?*
I keep them in one room there I got in my house, one special room for the bags—boxes, you know...I do my bags four times a day—in the morning about 6, one at 11, one at 4 and last one at 9 at night, you know.

And you never miss any?
No! [*laughing*] Doing real well!

Do you feel good now?
Yeah, I feel good; before—when I first came back from Perth—I used to drink too much water, tea, you know, and I was getting over—[loaded], eh? And I got short wind—you know, out of breathing—and they had to send me back again to Perth, and the doctor told me not to drink too much, you know—just drink a little sip of water.

And then you did that?
[*laughing*] Yeah, I'm doing that now! Yeah, it's more better. I don't get sick no more.

Like how much can you have—like a cup of tea, how much?
About half a cup in the morning and [again at] lunch time. I feel myself really good now if I don't drink much, you know. When I drink too much, I get too much fluid in my lung, you know—get short of breathing.

Yeah, I think that's a big problem for everybody. What about in the summer time?
Summer time, I'm right.

[*L.*:] It gets too hot in that room for you, though, doesn't it?

Yeah, it's a bit too hot.

You got any air conditioner?
No—but it's right when [the weather's] like this, you know, when it's overcast, you know—cool. When it's hot I get real no good inside, you know—too hot for me and I want to drink cold water every minute! [*laughs*] But when it's cold like this—it's a real beautiful day—I don't drink much then. When it's cold like this I can walk, you know, but when it's hot—it gets too hot for me [to walk]; I get all puffy, you know. In the winter time [it's] all right; sometimes I walk down to the hospital there, and they have to run me back [*laughs*]—I tell them it's too hot for me to walk back, you know—and they bring me back.

[She would prefer to have a trained helper but, so far, it has not happened.]

And did someone train with you—like someone in your family?
No...I wanted to teach my daughter to do it, you know, but she didn't want to [*laughs*]...I said, 'If I'm getting tired, well you can do my—do it—you know, I'll just lay back on the bed,' and she said, 'No Mum, I might do the wrong thing!' She wanted to, but—[*laughs*]

Does she watch you now when you do it? Does she keep an eye on you?
Yeah.

But she didn't want to learn?
No. [*laughs*]

[C.X. has to do the treatment regularly without any interruptions. She keeps written records.]

Yeah, I got a special room, eh. One room on the other side [of the house] and I got all the boxes stacked up there.

And your grandkids don't go in there?
No. I lock the door when I do my tube—I hunt him out [*laughs*]. He's a little boy, he's a nuisance! [*laughs*]—he's gotta come in and muck around—I told him, 'Get out!' No, I keep them out of that room. He see all the bottles there standing up, you know, and my [glasses] he always go for that glasses and puttem on himself. 'Oh, bring my glasses back—you might break it!' I always chase him out.

And you have to weigh yourself?
Yes, I weigh 38 [kg]. Every morning I weigh myself after I drain my bag out—I weigh myself on my scale—and scale for weigh them bags, you know. I weigh myself and my weight comes to 38 every morning—sometimes it go right back to 35—sometime it goes right up to 40, 41—when I have too much fluid, you know. When I drained my fluid out it goes right back to 38.

You should be about 38?
Yeah, I should be 38 all the time.

And if you got 41 [kg], what do you have to do?
That's too much—I go to hospital, you know. They tell me not to drink too much—I got too much fluid in me, you know. And I have to do five bags a day then, if I have too much fluid—five—one over [the limit] drain my fluid out—go back [to the proper weight] then.

Do you have to write that stuff down?
Yeah, I have a little black book there [*laughs*] and I keep it all there: what bag [number, i.e. strength of solution] I put in...and how much fluid I get out I put down...

So that keeps you busy every day, I suppose?
Very busy, and I got to do it at the right times, you know.

[C.X. can't do as much as she used to.]

Do you think that people who live in the bush—[in] communities—they could do this kind of thing—would it be too hard?
Oh, it'd be all right—maybe—as long as their place is clean, eh? It's important you have to be in a clean place—so you can't get infected, you know, in your bag—in your tube.

So you think it might be a bit hard if they lived out in the bush?
Yeah, out in the bush [it's] a little bit hard. [That patient] went out, eh?

[*L.:*] Yeah—she's gone for a holiday.

She went to [community R.].

How did she go? By motorcar?

[*L.:*] Yes.

Took her bags with her?
[*L.:*] Yep, she took everything.

I'm frightened to ride a motorcar, going out bush, you know, anywhere, fishing—I'm frightened because of my tube, maybe bump-bump, you know. One time I went out for ride to Palm Springs out here—that's a gravel road, you know. I was in the front seat but the bump-bumps were making my tube run. It was a bit hurting too, you know. So I don't go out any more now.

So you don't go fishing or anything like that?
No, I stay at home...I can walk down town, you know.

[C.X. has reliable and accessible medical support in the local community. Her family helps at home.]

[*L.:*] Yes, [the staff at the training centre and hospital in Perth] talk to us a lot—they'll ring us up tell us how people are going and let us know the date that they're arriving and Perth will book them into the hostel, where everybody has been—where [S.] was when she first came [back]. So we know when they're coming back and Homeswest [public housing authority] is notified so priority housing is put in a few months beforehand. They talk a lot to us.

When they come back home do the patients get a lot of help from the services?
[*L:*] The doctor has to see the patients every month to have bloods done—we test their blood, check their blood pressure and weigh them, and then we are in contact with them for ordering stock. But we only see people if they want to see us—if there's problems. Because by the time you get back, [*addressing C.X.*] you mob are so well trained—really well trained—that they come in and they settle down. I think it's scary for the first little bit—a bit frightening—but once people settle in, they don't need us—except for check-ups. We have to see them once a month, but that's all—and check the tube.

*[*to C.X.:*] So you're happy?*
I can do my tube with my eyes shut [*laughs*]. I don't worry, I don't go round for sister or anybody to help.

Do you have to buy anything yourself?
No, L.'s mob come down and look at my stock, eh? Let me know when it's coming on Gascoyne truck—and [the carrier] bring it right here in my house—they bring it right up here; they put it on this verandah and I cart it in—later on—because my son-in-law do that for me [*laughs*].

[*L:*] That's a big job that, eh?

Yeah.

How would you feel about showing us the room that you have everything in? Would it be all right?

Yeah [*laughing*]. It's nice and tidy—yeah—it's locked!

You have to watch your step all the time

We met B.L. in the Kimberleys. He is a Walmajarri man, born in the Gibson Desert. When we spoke at B.L.'s home, he had been back from Perth and in the community for three months. He spoke of how he manages (peritoneal) dialysis at home and then demonstrated an exchange for us.

I went to the dialysis first, on a machine, down Perth. It clean all the blood—the poison—right out...

So they asked you if you wanted to go on this [treatment]?
Yeah. When you out in the country, you have to have one of this [kind], you know, or if you want to stay on the machine, [then] you can go on the machine. But this one is a bit easier, you know, you knows how to handle it...That was bit hard for me on the machine, you know...

What do you think about this—do you think it's a good system?
Yep. This way is okay. Like you can do [it] at home—like what I'm doing here now. You can do it, you know—you have to watch your step all the time, on your dialysis like this...But [it's] right on the bag if they keep you in Perth [first]. They keep you in Perth till you well know this bag—really well—how to handle it. [You learn] how to do the bag...Before I went training [for] this, I went on the machine, then after, I [went] over there [to] the dialysis place, [to] learn this.

'Okay,' [the trainers] been tell me, 'you got to do your changing bag now.'

[T]hey stop there and watch me. They watch me there how I do it.

'Uh uh!—you [are] doing the wrong thing there—put this thing back on. [That's] how you start it first.'

'Oh yeah, sorry,' [I said].

Then I go again, then. And they watch you do all that thing—when you changing your bag you mustn't talk or anything, you know.

Concentrate?
Yeah, concentrate...otherwise...[?germs] from your voice—might go into your bag—bugs and things. [You have to] keep your table clean, like that—it's not good now [*the table had things spread over it*]. You're not allowed to have anything on your table, you only have—on the table—all your bag turnout [dialysis gear].

So when you start, you clear all that table down?
Yeah, clean all that, wash all that, with that [*indicating one of the bottles*]. Put my [dialysate] bag here; and all my clamps. Then go out [to] my bathroom—wash the sink down, hands [get] wash, and everything like that. When you emptying that bag...you go in the toilet and puttem down there. [Then] I just sit down here, I go to sleep if I want to...

One bloke haddem like this [CAPD] before me, you know—he never listened to the doctor when he told him—how you gotta do this and this—[how to] handle [the treatment] the proper way, you know...he's pass away now—he was a good young fella.

Mmm...yeah, that's the thing, [you've] got to be concentrating all the time.
Yeah, concentrating properly, and what[ever the] doctor tell you, you know, [if you do that] you're right—or dialysis [unit mob]—you got to listen when they tell you: 'Do it like this.'

You know—[if you take the catheter] just straight out—[say] he don't wash his fingernail or [something], you know—you got to be careful with that. [You've got wash your fingers] all this, all inside and here, here, here. [*B.L. demonstrates thorough hand cleaning, under the nails, between the fingers.*] Round everywhere—everywhere—every time...

[T]his [treatment is] all right, but [only] if a training [is] really good—very good, you know. They have to know very well for this; [it's a] bit dangerous this bag—you got to well know it, right through...

And what did you first think of this when you seen this bag? Did it make you frightened or—
Yeah, made me frightened...I thought [I'd have to] have this bag all the time, carrying it—this thing—all the time. Oh, I didn't like that! [*laughs*]

[There is a set pattern every day and B.L. has to be on the watch for signs of problems.]

...I do my bag, 7 o'clock this morning and 11 o'clock and 4, and 10 o'clock before I go to bed...four hours. See, I'm on a—like, too much weight now. I'm doing my [strong solution] bags, to get all my weight down.

Because you got too much at the moment?
Yeah, too much at the moment. I'm doing my [strong solution] bag. For a week—must be tomorrow, my sister [the nurse will] come along and check up [for] the dialysis centre and maybe my weight's going down...

Do you get tired of this, do you get sick of it sometimes?
Nah, nah. [*laughs*]

No? You just keep going?
Yeah, keep going...That's what I'm doing now—putting my weight down there [*showing his record book*]. [My] weight's over—76 [kg]—here somewhere [*following his records*]...They're all too high—too high, all the weight there.

What's the right one—what should you be?
I should be 72 [kg], somewhere round there...75 [is] too much.

Does somebody ever look in this book?
Yeah, my [nurse]—works at the [local] community health—they come and check me every Thursday.

If you got bag like this, it's okay now. You can see your finger right through—you can see my finger like that [*showing his hand clearly visible through the bag that's just drained*]; you can see it clear. Then that's a good bag...[If] you got a cloudy bag, that's no good for you.

Then what do you do?
You got to ring up to—you have to take them [bags] to the hospital. Take them to the hospital and ring the dialysis mob. See, I got all my phone [information] here, telephone number and all that—like they give me this one [*showing the papers from the dialysis unit*]. [It's] all here [*pointing out the numbers*]. Yeah, that's all the dialysis [numbers], and that's where I get all my gear.

Did that problem ever happen?
I had [it] one time. Yeah, I had my bags—like really cloudy. That's infected inside [your body], you know. You have to take your bags straight in there [local clinic] and they give you needle on that other bag—[the] new bag [the clinic puts antibiotics into the dialysate].

They take it [the catheter] out and open this [cap] up and put a needle inside here. Antibiotics, you know—[you have to] leave it [in] there for six hours—then you drainem out again...

And the next one was clear for you that time?
Yeah...and then I start all over again. If you keep on [having the problem] like that, well they take you down to Perth.

[He had to leave his old house when he started on this treatment. He has a new house in town now, but that has brought some extra problems.]

They been give me this house [because] I had this problem.

Where did you live before?
At the reserve down there...Yeah—just old humpies and houses. I been living on that little humpy and they asked me for [said I needed] a house. No house out there. [But I needed] a good house...They been find out I come back and they been give me house then. See, you need a good house to do all your bag here; you need a good running water and all that, you know—

You didn't have any running water before—where you were living before?
Ahh, yeah, [it was a] bit rough and ready...

You mustn't talk to any people [like this:] 'Come in'—like [inviting] drunken people—come into your house and—you know.

Is that a problem for you—or that's all right?
Ahh, that's a big problem there. You have to hunt them people away, you know, or call the police. You know, like I'm here, [if] all my people come here—come drunk or anything—I have to call the police to come and—

Is that a bit hard for you?

Yeah, a bit hard for me, like—you know—have to hunt them away, you know. I tell them not to come here, you know...

Do those people—they know you got this [treatment to do]?
Yeah, they know.

[He has taken one trip out to his home outstation.]

Can you travel around a bit or you got to stay here in one place?
Yeah, you can—you can travel around, you know. Long as you have everything and all your gear's up there. You can travel round—where you want to go, you can go.

And you been any trips, you been anywhere?

Yeah, I went out there to the community—my community.

And you took this, all this here?
Yeah, I took six—six of them—six bag of 2 [strength solution] and six of 1 [strength solution].

And how long did you stay out there?
Just for, ah, for weekend, you know, like went on Friday and come back on Sunday.

Right—no problem?
Nah, no problem. Long as you have to have a clean place to do your changing, bag and like that. Same thing like—you got a community out there with a clinic, you know...[w]ell anybody can change [their] bag in the clinic—in a clean place, there...

If I want to move anywhere, I can go...like go for a holiday somewhere, well, then you have to ring up to your place, to your boss [at the dialysis unit], well, they send you all that—bags and everything, 'cause you have to take it when you move, you know.

Could you live out at [community W.]?
Oh, yeah, [but] it's hard—it's [a long way] out from this place, it's bit too rough country, you know. No good for coming in [to Fitzroy Crossing], only [and] sometime rain—never come out—you know [i.e. might get rained in at the community]...There's a clinic there...[but] I like to be close to this hospital there, you know.

[It seems as if B.L. has to forgo his involvement in the major religious ceremonial activity of the region. He can no longer join countrymen travelling across the desert on business.]

We [Walmajarri and Pitjantjatjara people] got a same language. See, we all come from desert—all from Gibson Desert and they all spread out; 'nother mob went that way, all other [mob] went this way, Kalgoorlie side—same language.... Walmajarri is different language from this area [here]—Fitzroy area...[but] all our desert people can talk the same language from Balgo right up to Territory...

So you travelled around this desert country a bit, eh?
Yeah—no [not just travelling] we travelled around with the law time, you know—every law time.

Which way you travelled down through?
Out in the South Australia area...Warburton language...Blackstone—all that area.

You think you'll be able to go with this gear?
No, I can't go with this. No—too far with this...I can't go. I used to go long time [i.e. before], but not now—[I] can't really. You can't go past the community out there—about 80 km from here—that's [how] far you can go.

Sometime family givem a hard time

M.N. and A.S. head a household on one of Alice Springs' town camps. At the time of this interview they had two renal patients, and their respective partners, living within their extended household. They gave their thoughts on why patients miss sessions on the dialysis machines. They answer with reference to the patients they know.

M.N.: [L.Y., a patient] run to me and she tell me, 'My husband give me hard time!'

And I tellem that old man, 'Don't givem hard time! She gotta go to [dialysis] machine.'

I gavem [gave her] that $20 and I puttem in that taxi now, and she went to the machine. And I been tellem [that husband], 'Don't worry—she'll come back home. You go and drink around—but she got no-good two kidneys—you right [to go yourself now]. Saturday and Sunday—machine not working—[so she'll have the] weekend off. She gotta go one time now—Friday—[to] that machine.'

A.S.: But this [treatment]: they got to go *all* the time, see, all the time—not to miss one day or two day—they got [to] keep going all the time. But [there's] a problem up here sometime, [their] family givem hard time—[her] husband givem hard time...[he] want [her] to stay here...[But, on the other hand, J.I., the other patient in their house] always go out with his wife—[he] can't leavem here.

M.N.: [He] always takem—to machine—and all the Whitefella from machine, they get angry, [saying,] 'You don't bring [your] wife to machine, you got to come by [your]self!'

Why can't he take his wife there?

M.N.: Too much taking [her] everytime...[She's] getting sick of it every time. They [the staff] seen that a lot of time...some [staff] get sick of it—only they want 'kidney people'—[the] 'no kidney' people, that's all [i.e. only patients are welcome].

A.S.: [But] he worrying that someone might take his wife away.

That's why he's got to takem over there?

A.S.: *Yuwayi* [yes]. Someone might take his wife away [*laughs*].

M.N.: But [his wife] she been tell me, 'I been sitting down there all day and waiting! [So] I ran away in the taxi.' Too much sitting for her [*laughing*]. [Her] husband givem hard time...[he] always go out with his wife...he can't leavem here [at home].

[*They note wider family problems associated with urban living.*]

A.S: Hardest thing for him to live [here is] because he got a family [that] gives him hard time, 'specially the son—you know when [he] live in town—he get hard times.

M.N.: The son get drunk and give him a hard time—[the] father...But they want to stay with family—make [them] happy, you know.

A.S: [Before], he used to stop in Sid Ross Hostel...

M.N.: When they staying in a hostel they really boring [i.e. isolated]—you [need to] stay close family, like [in the] Aborigine way.

Lonely—year after year

The following interview was conducted with R.N., a renal patient, on the lawns in front of her hostel. R.N. lives there alone. Her family were at a distant community. She listened briefly to an explanation of the purpose of the research, but shortly interrupted and began speaking about her situation.

People can't stay away from their families. They got no money to come down here [Alice Springs], it's a real problem. I need families to stay with me—I'm always by myself.

Does anyone from your family come here to stay?
Sometimes my husband comes for two days and goes back—they not used to town.

What about brothers or sisters?
My brothers and sisters don't come. Sometimes I get lonely, you know, [and then] I take up with any car. When I was really sick I was doing that, [I] used to get a lift with any car. The doctor got really upset, bit worried. I was running from here to home.

Did the doctor growl [reprimand] you?
No, they can't. Now I'm getting good now, going on the plane. I go Tuesday and come back Friday, go on the machine on Saturday.

What did your family say when you ran away from here?
They was upset. They told me, 'You shouldn't run away from hospital!' And I told them, 'I'm getting homesick, I need family to stay with me.'

[At this point in the interview R.N. became upset; she turned away and started crying. For about ten minutes she sat with her back turned towards the interviewer, not saying anything, but wiping her eyes from time to time. The interview began again at R.N.'s instigation with a question about two other women patients who were also living at the hostel.]

I don't know them—a lot of strange people here. [*R.N. regained her composure and shifted around to face the interviewer again.*] I don't like to talk about my kidney problem 'cause I got no one here with me. We need a machine in our community, we can't sit down lonely year after year...

[The interviewer raised the possibility of her getting work as an interpreter because her English is good.]

Yes, I like to do work, not to wander around here—get homesick and worry too much.

i had a family that talked to me

In 1987, before dialysis was available in Alice Springs, patients had to relocate to Adelaide for treatment. C.L., a renal patient who had spent time in Adelaide, told his story—part of which is reproduced below—on video, to encourage other patients. For him, family support is the key to his perseverance.

You see it's a hard thing for Aboriginal people to come in from communities without their family—the first thing they look for is a brother...Or a [town] camp, it's the first place they go, it might be a tin shack, but it's still a home away from home.

I was lucky. I had a family that talked to me—my eldest son, my daughter, my wife. I wanted to throw it in. That's the way I felt—being hooked up to a machine. I thought, 'I'm halfway there, why not go all the way?' They coaxed me, walked me around, gave me exercise, walked me around the block, went in the sun. Seeing that gave me hope. Someone has some love for me. A lot of people from Alice came down to Adelaide to see me. Well, that gave me new hope. Well, I thought, 'Right! If they're there for me, then I'm there for them.'

I got that weak [on dialysis], I was going to come home to Alice Springs and chuck it in. [The family] stayed with me right through, brought me right back. One of my grand-daughters—[she's] about twelve—from the day I went with my family she stayed until the day I came back. Today she's a very happy girl.

If someone is on the machine and really wants to get back into the real way of life—I nearly threw it in—don't ever think about that because there's always hope. Our doctors today—they're magic. I still tell people, 'They could take this part out of the next person and put it into you, away you go!' That's why I'm sitting here telling the people: 'If you've got a chance to get a transplant kidney—go for it! Don't be frightened!' Take notice of your doctor. Every day you come to the machine, think about that. Take your drugs if they tell you; if you miss a couple of times, your blood might change from the other person. The right one will check—there it is: new life!

I'll tell you what, after being on a machine, you [will] get around like I do. I'm back to doing a bit of light work...I feel 100% better. My family doesn't have to cart me around as they did when I was on the machine. Things I had to watch, eat, drink, stick to my tablets. It's back to normal life.

I think to have a transplant kidney is one of the greatest things that's ever happened to me after how weak and ill I was. Not being hooked to a machine. The main thing is take notice of your doctor. Do what he tells you and stick to the rules—the guidelines. That's the main thing.

Stick with it, don't give up hope! Think of the other people out there trying to help you...

I'm glad they were there to help me.

(Excerpt from 'Renal Video' made by Territory Health Services, Alice Springs, 1994)

they put up with it

Renal patients sometimes find themselves extremely isolated. Without their usual wide family support network, patients may find it difficult to change unacceptable situations or challenge those who are causing them problems. A family member describes the situation she came across while visiting her sister on dialysis in Alice Springs.

And then they stayed at House Two [on a town camp]—oh terrible!...Nobody's giving them support in home management, anything like that. [Why don't they] just give them a bit of support there, you know? Clean the house, do a bit of shopping, get them to organise themselves, budgeting, that sort of thing, you know. I think it is really hard, because when I went down to see [her] there, she couldn't do any shopping or anything, she had no vehicle at that time and [her husband] was drinking and people were going into their room and taking things that was 'specially for her, you know. She put up with a hell of a lot of problems.

Did she complain to you?

Uh uh [no]. I could see it myself—and I ended up slamming two of the women there in her yard!

[T]hey come in there drunk and they're trying to push sick people around—and they were all dialysis patients the ones that were staying with her. [That woman], she's drunk—she goes to them, pushes them around—wants tobacco, wants this, you know, saying really abusive things to them. I don't know [what my sister did about it], she never told us anything, but I ran into [the drunken woman] a couple of times and the second time around, I gave it to her! She made me really sick! I couldn't take it for those sick people—what they go through—they can't put up with that sort of thing all the time.

She don't go round there now, because [my sister's] husband stopped drinking too—they don't let any drunks go there now. But before, what about the [patients] that have drunken people going in there terrorising them in their homes and taking off with their food and stuff: that's what needs to be addressed, I think. That's why a lot of people don't stay in Alice Springs, because they got no security in their homes—no sort of support and security. Maybe a couple of people should go round every day just to see how they're going—if they've had any problems. [My sister] had to put up with all that first—and she was really sick and weak, you know, when we came up from Adelaide.

But she never said anything?

No.

Why do you think that is—that people put up with that kind of stuff?

They put up with it because they're sick and they don't want to get hurt—especially the dialysis patients. They say, 'Oh well, I better not say a thing out of line otherwise I'll be [knocked] down, you know and I'll be in more worse condition than what I am now'— they think [to] themself. They have got no family there [in Alice Springs] to support them—that's why I think somebody should go around and support them—see what things they need and just help them, because they're on their own—they got no families [in Alice Springs]. And a lot of the family members don't want to go down to Alice. What about in the future, they are going to have dialysis machines put up here, set up here in this hospital or what?

We can't rubbish them

Three women who are renal patients discuss the way family relationships are important to them and cause them so much worry.

How do your families feel about missing out on family business—like sorry business and that kind of thing?

W.S.: [My family said] not to go and travel round for young fella [business] and finish-off [business], they told us to stay here. They got a bit of sense, you know; sick people not allowed to come here at wrong place and come and cry—they might make theirself more sick—that's what they said, they don't worry about us, you know. They don't get cranky. They told us [that] we can't go when we sick—while we on the machine. That what they told me—all my family. 'No,' they said, 'that's all right you can stay [in Alice Springs] because you're sick, you can stay [there] close to machine, don't worry about it.'

But I got worry from here. I was very very sad, trying to go and finish-off, but I went there and she was gone. That's why I stayed there and come back Sunday night—

T.N.: —yeah, them family can say it's all right for us not to go down there, you know, but sometimes it's *us*, you know, *we* have feeling—how *we* feel—we got to go still. It's like me, I still want to go back there, still go and share sorrow with our family, you know, show them that we still care for them, you know, think about them—never mind we too far.

O.S.: Mmm...

T.N.: We can't rubbish them—show our back [to] them. And like business, especially corroboree time—it's good fun that one—it's the time we come together, you know, [to] enjoy—enjoy everything—dancing—sometimes we see men's dancing, [sometimes] women's. You know, we still got to go back and look back at our culture even though we're living here. We still got to go back—we can't just live here, eh?...I like to go back one day—back up there—but I just can't go. Like maybe [I can] get a transplant quickly or—I don't know—or talk to them to give us that other sort of thing [CAPD].

O.S.: [*translated from Warumungu*] Yes, when I go back [home] my family tells me, 'You'd better go back.' They send me back [to Alice Springs] quickly. 'You go back closer to the machine. Don't keep coming back here, or you might get worse.' My children get anxious and they send me back: 'Don't stay here for a week, or two weeks.'

And that's why I always go Friday, Saturday and Sunday, come back...They can't forget [me]—they always hunt me back—[make me] come back. They always tell me, 'Mum, you're gotta go back because you might get really sick.'

i'll be walking around for fishing

A renal patient, R.S., has haemo-dialysis at her home in a small town in the Kimberleys. Her grandson, S., and her niece have been trained to operate the dialysis machine which is set up in one room in her home. They help each other to carry out the treatment three times every week and have been doing this for the last four years. R.S. and her two partners talk about how they manage.

R.S.: No, I didn't want the bag—they took me in [and] they showed me—I been look at the machine, and the bag, they showed me, and they said, 'Which one do you want, the machine or the bag?'

So then I ask them, 'How many hours [is] the bag?'

'Oh, every four hours, you know.'

Every four hours! You can't go anywhere—you gotta be all the time home, you know—you can't visit your people or anything like that on the weekends and things like that. So I said, 'I'll go on the machine.' So I went on the machine then.

I didn't like the bag. They were saying [things] like the bag was danger for me, you know, I got grandkids and things like that—little ones [that might be] jumping on my tummy, and like that, you know...my tube might come out—that's why I was frightened—so I asked them for the machine...They was going to put me [and the machine] at the [local] hospital. I said, 'I want my machine at home, you know, close—this is my home, here.'

[R.S. and her two partners had to be trained in Perth.]

R.S.: When we down to Perth...and they didn't take me long to get trained, you know.

S.: Yeah, for about three months we went down there. But we had one other machine before this. We went down [to Perth] and trained for it—for about three months, then we came back and later on we switched onto this [newer] one. [R.S.] had the machine there at the dialysis centre in Perth, and they showed us how to operate [it] there—in that hospital. Once we knew how to set it up and everything, we came back this way then and they installed one here in this house.

They come back with you?

S.: Oh yeah. [They stayed] only for one night.

R.S.: We had the books and everything.

S.: There's a book [illustrated manual] there, it shows you how to set up the machine and everything. When we first started—[we were] very nervous! We got used to it, then we didn't worry about it much then. It was just all right with us.

What's the main things you have to be careful of?

S.: The main things? Her weight—how much fluid you taking out of her; when you take out fluid from her body, you have to be sure how much you taking out—'cause if you take out too much she'll start getting cramp...[It's] not really [hard]—once you get the hang of it; you don't worry about it.

R.S.: You got to keep it clean, you know—when you finish—you just chuck all this one away [*indicating the machine tubing*].

S.: When she comes off, we just get all these blood lines and just chuck them in the bin...All that rubbish—that thing there, they all go up to the hospital.

And who has to do that?

R.S.: Oh—sometime we takem back. They have to go to Derby, all that stuff you know...all the blood line and thing, they go in that rubbish bin there.

When you run out of the stores [or] get low, you got to ring Perth up, and letting them know. [You must] keep your stores up, you know—everything.

S.: Yeah, all the three of us do [the ordering. The order] comes straight here.

R.S.: [By] truck, yeah—comes straight here.

[R.S. explained how she manages her treatment and fits it into her life.]

R.S.: Well, say if I have long weekend like Saturday and Sunday off, if I drink too much water or tea, I can feel that fluid inside and I gotta stop and be careful. And sometime I got to get [S.] up late at night or late in the afternoon or something like that, could be three hours just to take that fluid out. I feel all right after that. And next morning after that three hours, I can go two hour and that makes the five hours, see?

So, like [the day after the session] you'll feel good?

R.S.: I must [only] have a little bit of meat...or light [meal] or eggs or something like that. Not really meat with the fat and thing like that. You got to be very careful for your kidney, you know—and for your heart. If you get fat and things like that—and [your] heart will be that big [*indicating size*]. Half a cup of tea, or if you want a slice of bread or something like that, and meat—little bit of meat.

[And] vegies—what I do, sometime I just eat the raw one, like cabbage—cut the cabbage up or lettuce or something, but...if you have boiled cabbage or something like that—[and leave] all the water, still in the cabbage...that fill you up inside. You got to be very careful with your fluids. You got to check with your dry weight and your fluids.

S.: [That red folder there,] that's her chart.

R.S.: [My] chart for the weight and thing like that—blood pressure.

S.: Weight and blood pressure, that's what [we] always do there—before she goes from [this room]. Before she goes on, we do her weight and her blood pressure and even when she comes off [we do it again].

R.S.: And the weight drops down.

So you'll be up and around tomorrow?

R.S.: Yeah, I'll be walking around for fishing or anything like that or shopping or anything like that. Wednesday morning [my grandson], he'll be off, the lady will come around—[my] niece.

Feel good, sometime—sometime I feel...umm...tired, you know, from the machine. Sometime I'm right, I can walk around, then we go fishing and thing like that. [Sometimes] I go bush...I might go weekends somewhere in the 'nother place and I come back on Sunday.

[R.S. places the needles in her own arms at the beginning of the session. The carer helps.]

S.: She does [the needles] by herself—do it by herself.

R.S.: You can't feel it or anything, you know, but you...got to do it by—if you gonna push or something like that, you got to hold, you know.

S.: She did that first on the little one—the little needles—and that makes it [her arm] numb—then she put the other two—see them ones there in the box there—she puts the little needle...and then...puts those two in—one here and one here—arterial and the venous—and see from here where it's connected—that's how long [the needles] are and that's connected onto the machine.

[The group are ready to deal with problems and have an excellent support network.]

We just ring up down to that home dialysis down in Perth [Royal Perth Hospital] there. We just ring up down there and like they tell us what to do over the phone. We just tell them, like, if it's the heparin pump or anything like [that]; if the red light is still on. They'll just tell us over the phone.

R.S.: Like if I get sick or anything like that, or if I get short wind or anything like that, I got the oxygen there.

Did you have to go back to Perth at all—you had any problems?

R.S.: No, no. I just go there for the check-ups.

How often do the technicians come up here?

S.: Comes about once a month [from Perth]...We come over and watch. There's a man and woman technician—Cheryl and Fred.

R.S.: Yeah. Then the lady [nurse] from [the local] community health—Sister Joy—[s]he come up every Thursday—fill all the dosette box. Every Thursday, got to bring all the tablets. I always puttem all the tablets [myself]. [You] make sure you got to leave that cramp tablets out—you might get cramp. I had the bed here [and] I used to get cramp every day on the bed, but the chair there better, you know—you can put your leg down if you want to rest it.

[The two partners (carers) have to think ahead as well.]

And how did you get this job?

S.: I volunteered for it. Yeah, me and [the other woman] did. In 1991 we went down to Perth to train how to do this.

And how long you been doing it now?

S.: From 1991, yeah, four [years]...Like if I want to go somewhere, I tell [R.S.'s niece, the other carer]—and she'll do it...when I'm supposed to, [then] when I come back I'll do it while she's going on holidays. She went to Melbourne for Christmas holiday and she went for three weeks and I did it for three weeks here and when she came back, I had my three weeks off.

[Some people are not keen to learn to operate the dialysis machine.]

R.S.: Some people, they frightened. They asked two people from [a nearby community]—they got a relation down in Perth there—and they want [their] brother [to] coming here to watch [my grandson and niece]. Just a practising, you know—but they too frightened.

They say, 'Oh we don't want to do it.'

[The] blood frightened them. [If you've got ESRD] you got to have the machine [to] keep your body well so you don't die young or anything like that. They want couple of partners go [for training] but they don't want to come and watch these two doing it...they [potential partners] too frightened.

[The patient is] still down Perth. They sendem back last year to the community—to the old people's home—with the bag see—had a bag. She used to sneak away from the hostel there and wait there with the 'nother friends—he drive [her] around with the motorcar and they used to go sometimes drinking—when [she] had the bag.

[She describes others who have returned with dialysis machines and not managed so well.]

R.S.: Other two friend of mine—they died now—they had the machine up at the hospital there. They used go down to the hospital every [day]. What happened [was] they never been looking after theirself. [They would] go home and never have a bogey—wash their arm before they put your needle in. You got to wash your arm—and get all your tray ready, [get] all the things set up—all your needle. But those two old ladies never look after theirselves, you know.

Did they have their carers with them?

R.S.: Yeah, the one lady had the two daughter, and 'nother one had daughter, and sister. But they used to go down the pub drinking and

How do the relatives, doctors
nurses, etc.
understand the renal
patient? the treatment,
the machine

p 52
Argue that "on the
other hand there is a
driving compulsion to
escape the social &
cultural isolation of Alice
Springs –" but also
escape the Western notions
the machine??

see pp54 et foll

Kinship is not redefined
among patients? why?

"on the machine 4

- ≠ options
- home dialysis
  peri & haemo

On the machine 3

How are dr. machine &

staff separated?

patient versus non-patient –

∘ Machine makes you sick

sleep & you're better

∘ Not enough explanations

from doctors / both patients &

relatives complain →

obligation

family resp–

leave away from

community & respons–

becoming conscious of

"one's life, one's

body in ≠ ways

p18 "The machine"

"The sisters help make me better, looking after me every day, but you know it was only one thing — the Kidney machine — that really made me better — It wasn't a person who made me better — it was that machine"

p ~~21~~-23 sorcery / Kidney

p27 → strain (lots of)

→ get info on what people think about ≠ kinds of machines -

"On the machine" (1)

Communicating like a kin (a friend) Rewards (pp 5-6) "I feel happy, they feel happy"

ATSIC health

funding? for machines in communities?

Kidney pbls increase because of sugar, food 12-15 consumed today, medicine of today versus the white food & ngangayi / ngankari

[illegible] new. broken ⟹ 15-16

Wiradjuri

most often mentioned

causes = grog

i sorcery -

ill sugar

see p 78 - 79 →

"Respondents who provided 2 or more causes implied - though rarely spelled out - that these factors had combined in some way to produce disease."

---

elizabeth.edwards.pitt-rivers-museum.oxford.ac.uk

gaynor on Roviana art

then come back half hangover in the morning. [They] never used to do the right thing for the old lady, you know—and then [she] went home and—just passed away, yeah.

But the other one had the no-good liver...the last one [to pass away]...You can't have crowd of people in the house [on this treatment]. You might have two workers and [a] daughter whatever. [But say if you had] a husband—drunken husband—well you got to keep the husband away from the wife. You got to live [with just your] own family in the house—no drunks or anyone because otherwise they'll give you headaches and all that—you'll have lot pressure on you now.

That's not a problem for you here?

R.S.: No, no. They look after me...A friend of mine from Mt Barnett, he went down in Perth there—and he had the bag and when he went back to Derby, he start go down to the Reserve and thing like that. [He] had little bit of dinner and feed with relations—[his] daughter, son—they gave him little bit of drink [alcohol] and things like that, you know.

[The machine has to be carefully looked after.]

S.: If you got a good house and thing like that—good water—make sure you keep the house clean. But [you] got to be very careful of dust.

R.S.: They can have [the machine] in a home, long as they remember to cover the machine up with a sheet or something like that, so the dust can't get into it.

If they don't want to stop in hospital all the time—they want to go home [for] home dialysis—they got to keep it [the place] clean; keep your house tidy—wash the floor. [If] people got a big family—well you got to keep the [room] shut all the time because the kids—see those two, the little ones there—that's my grandkids, but the other one [has] gone to school. Now this one—might be two or three [years old]—she come here and play here, mucking around, [well] I just hunt them away. But they mustn't touch the machine, the kids—[they] might change him around and things like that. You got to keep the door locked. Little kids might be touching all that thing and this machine [will] go wrong.

Short stories about different kinds of treatment for kidney failure

- *on the machine*
- *a stranger's kidney*
- *the bag*
- *family way*

You can ask your health service more about these stories and this kidney sickness

On the machine

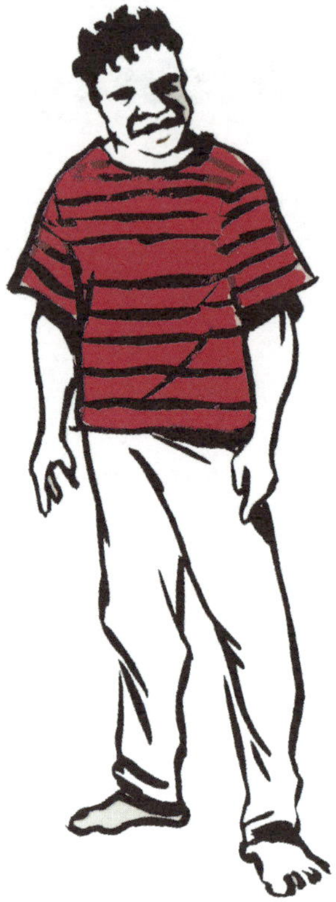

What happened to
Maxie

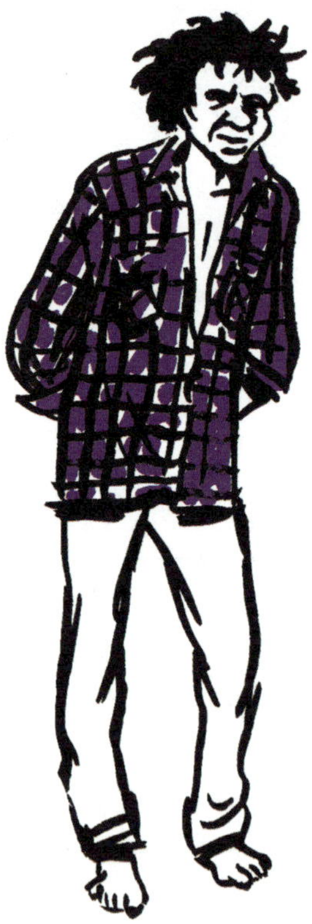

and Archie...

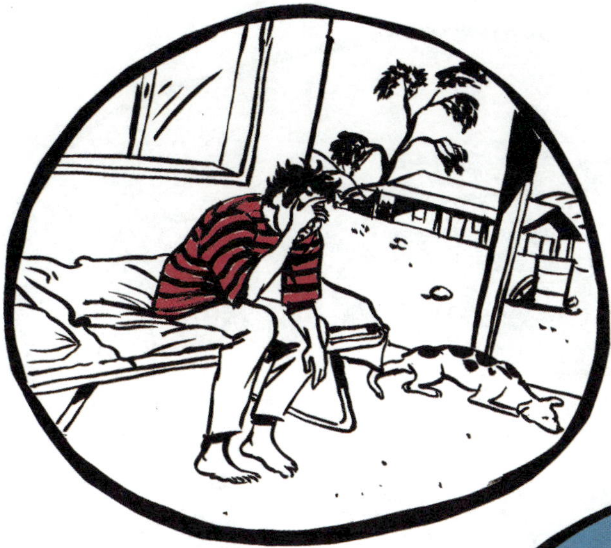

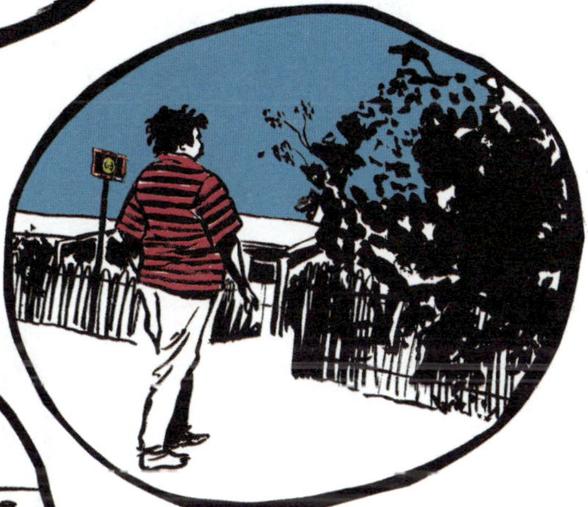

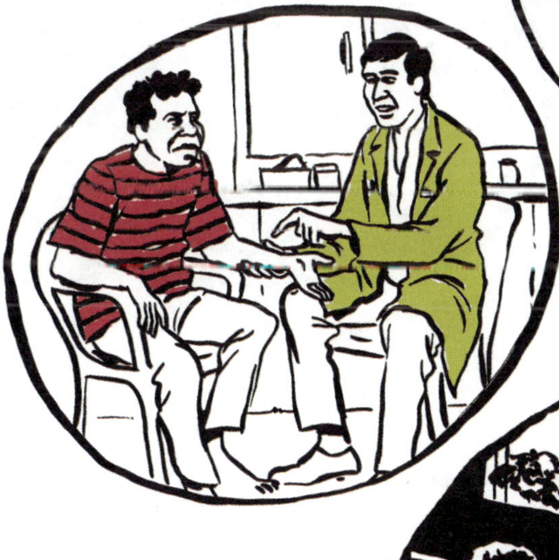

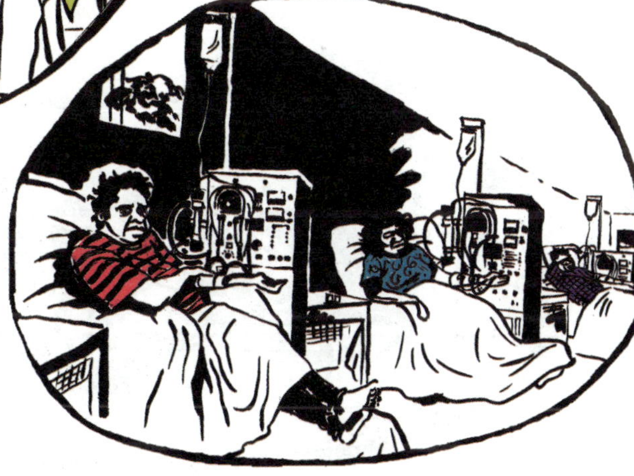

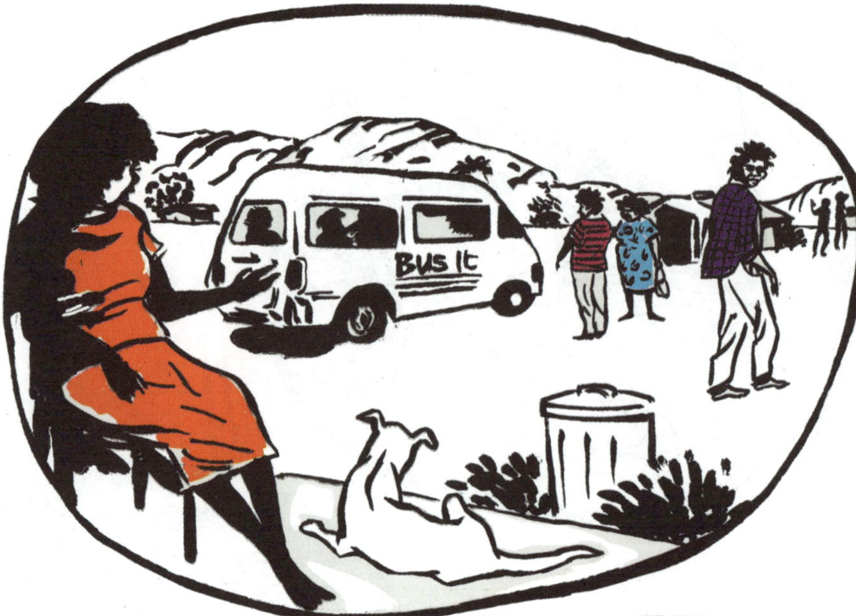
Bus It

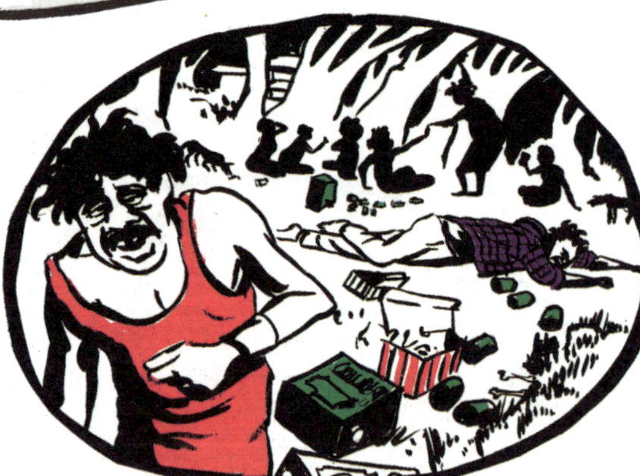

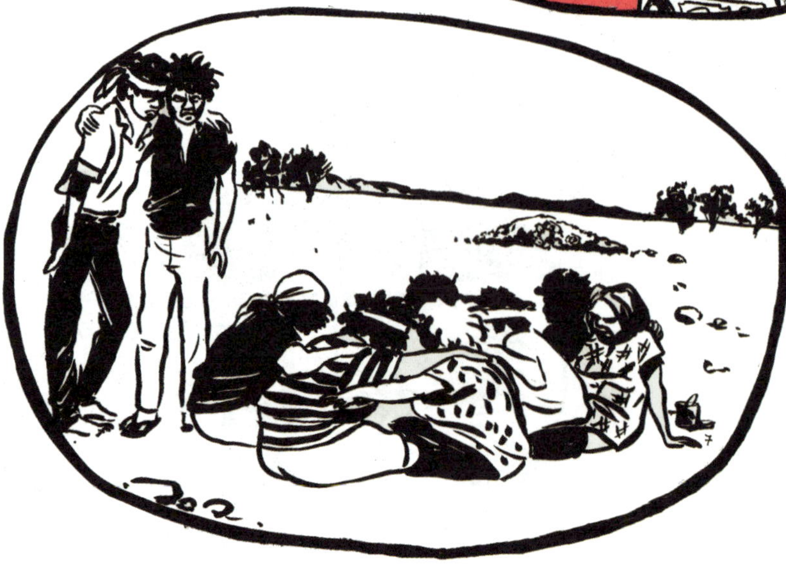

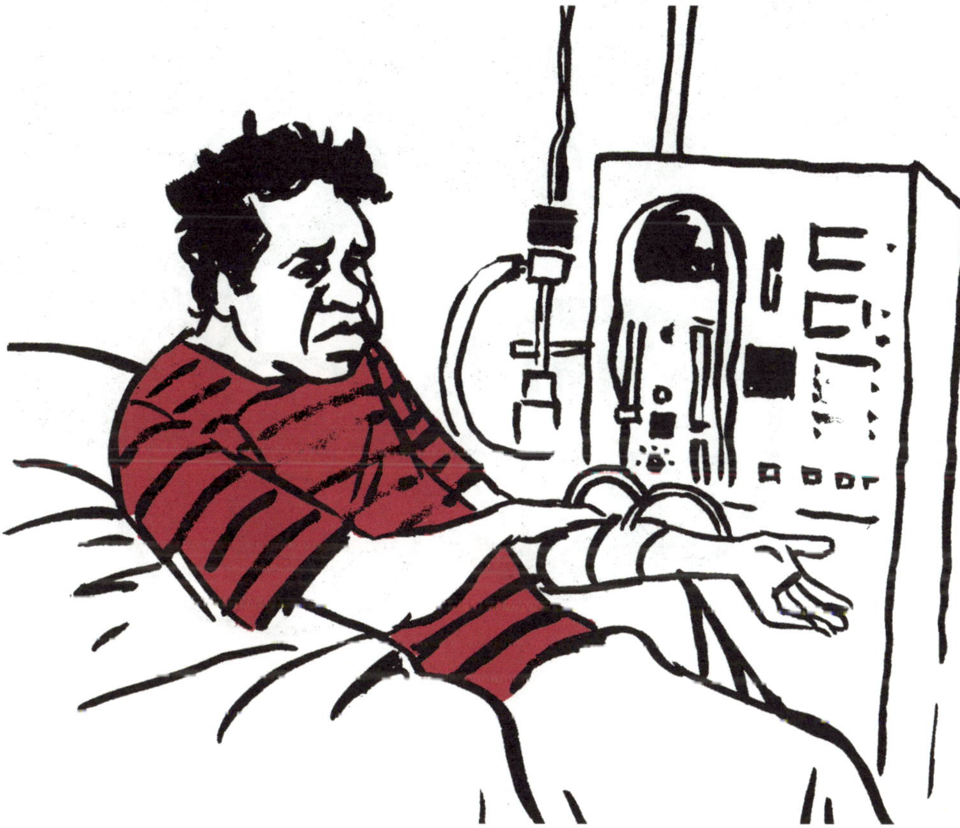

What happened to Maxie later...

in Adelaide a man was killed in an accident

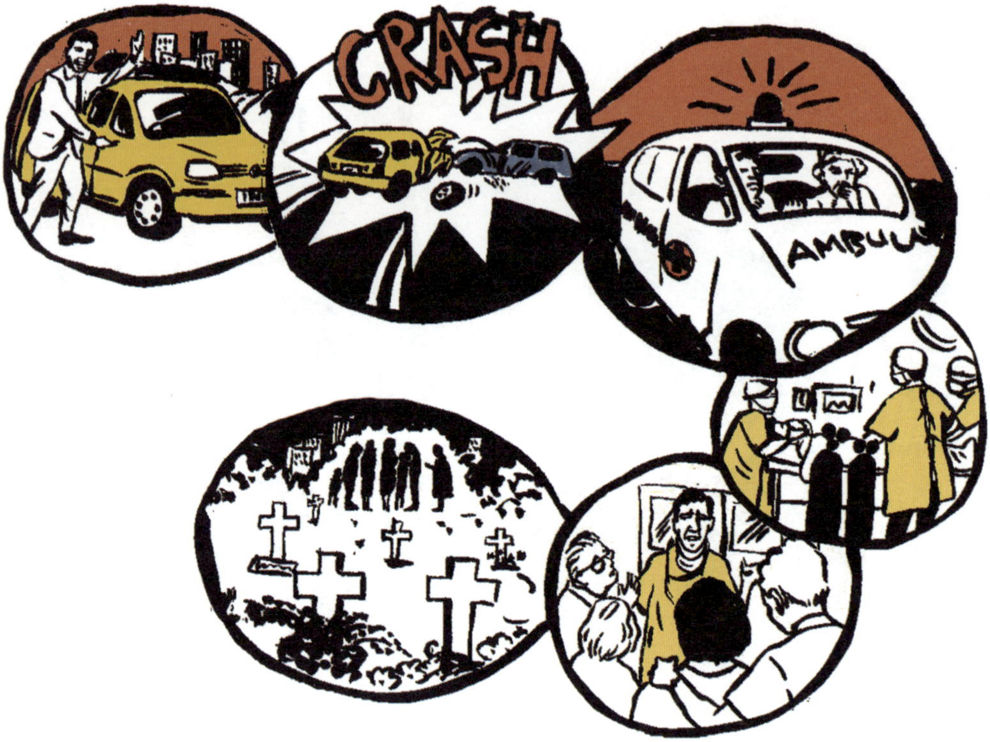

and his family gave his kidneys to the hospital.

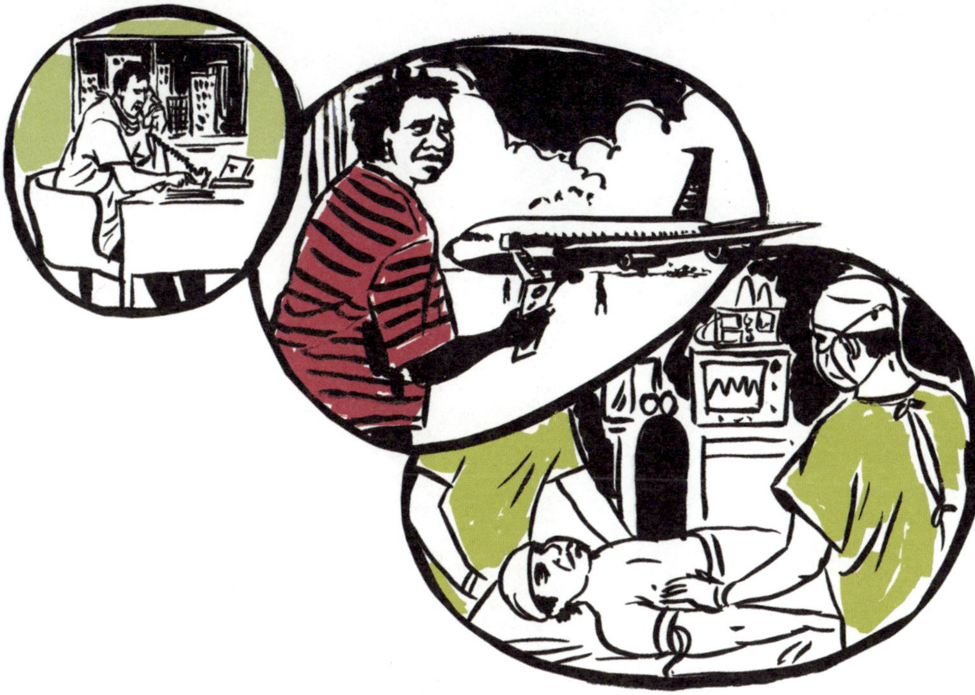

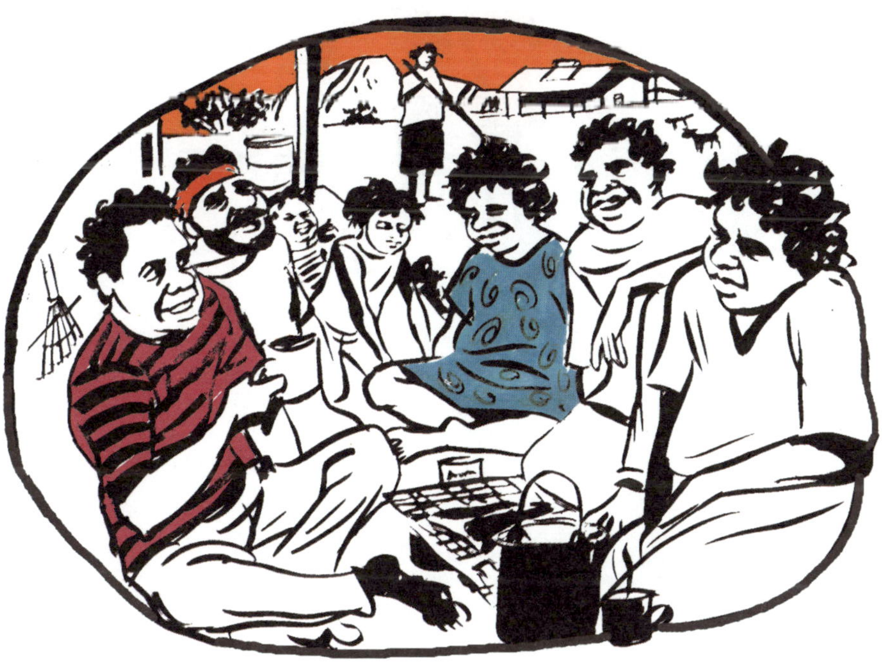

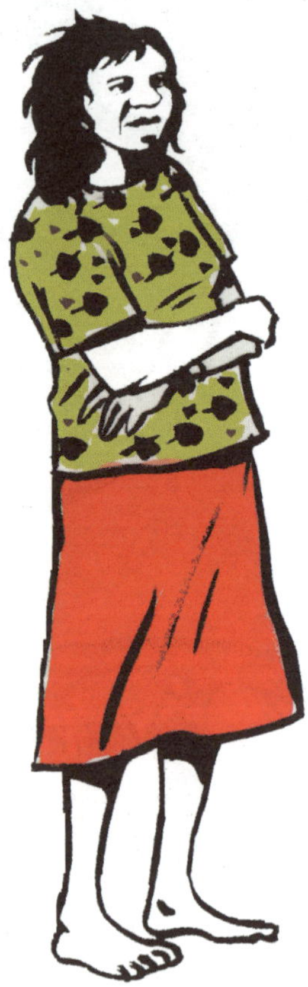

What happened to Vera...

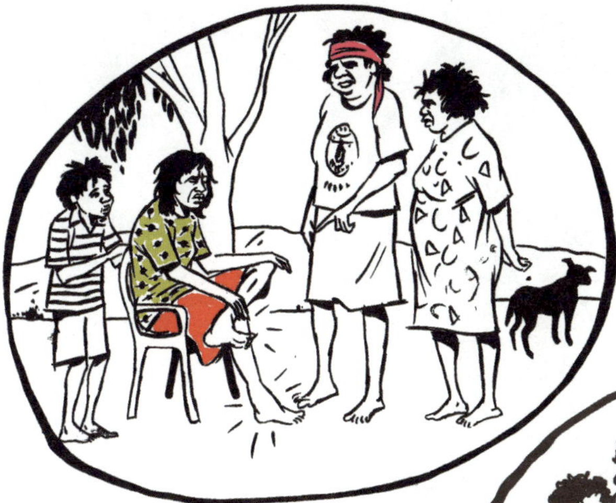

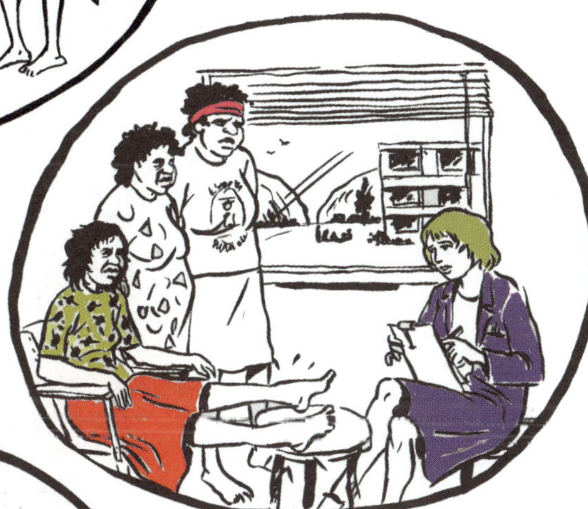

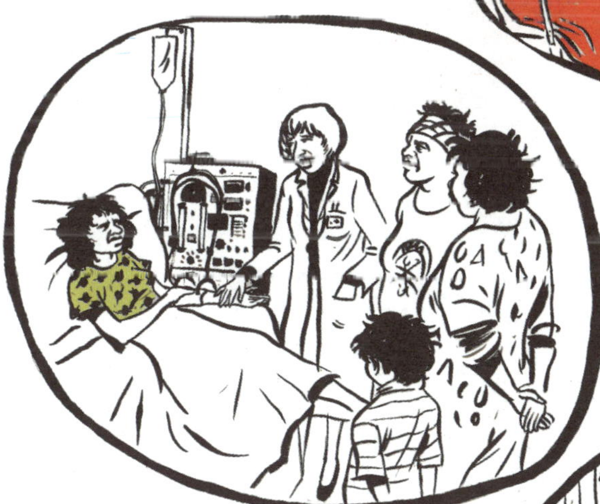

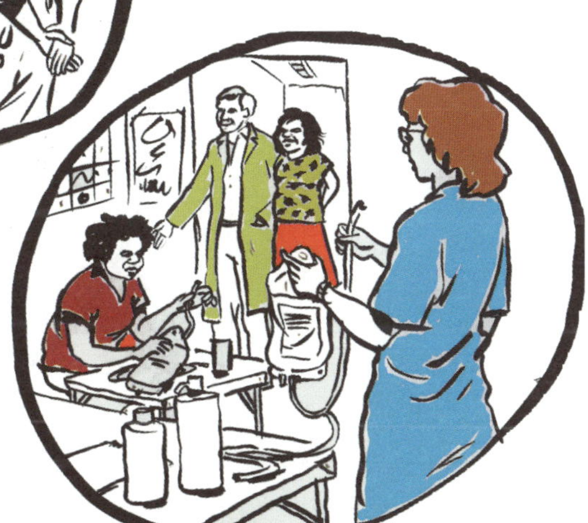

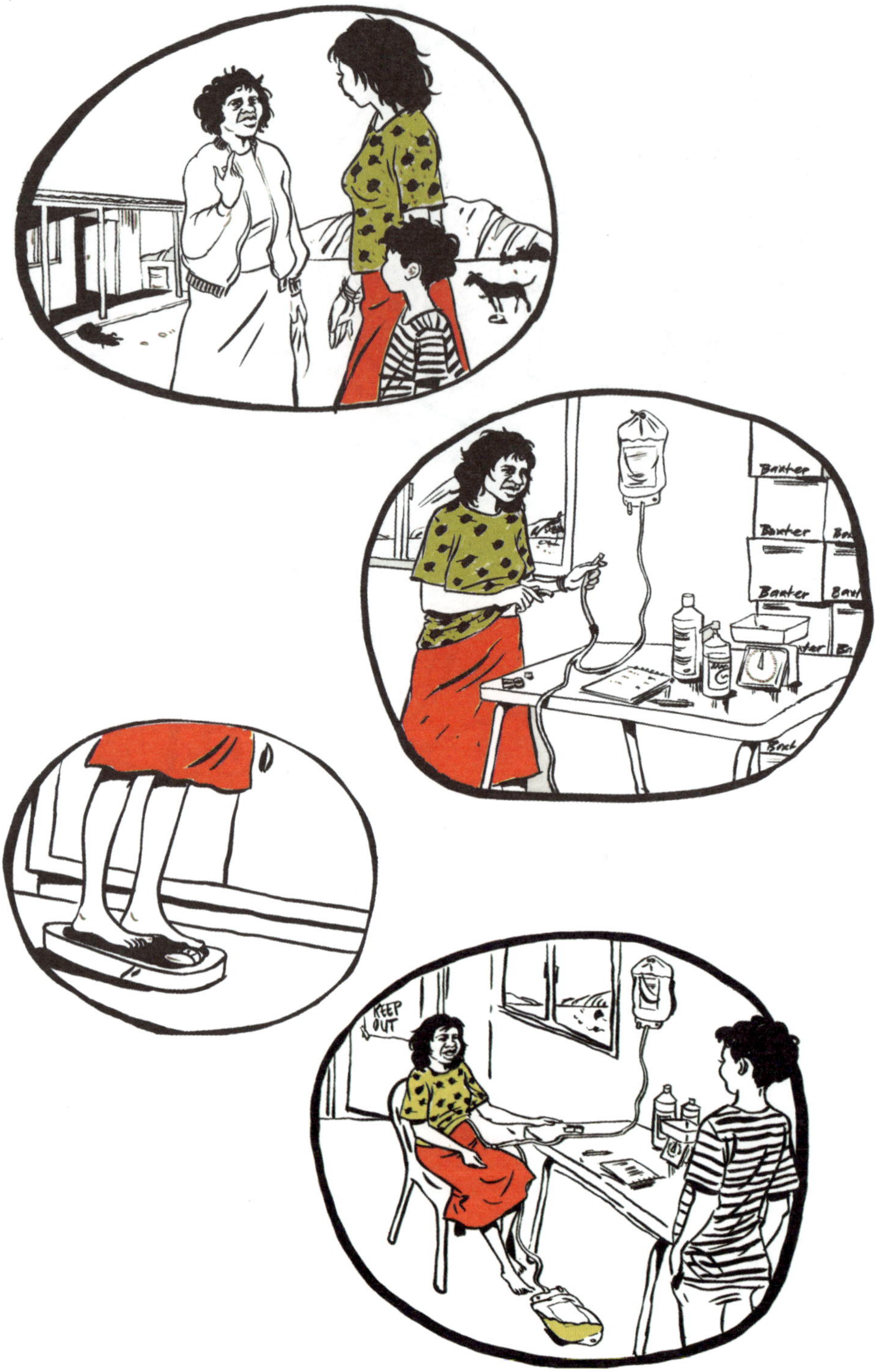
Baxter
Baxter
Baxter
KEEP OUT

family way

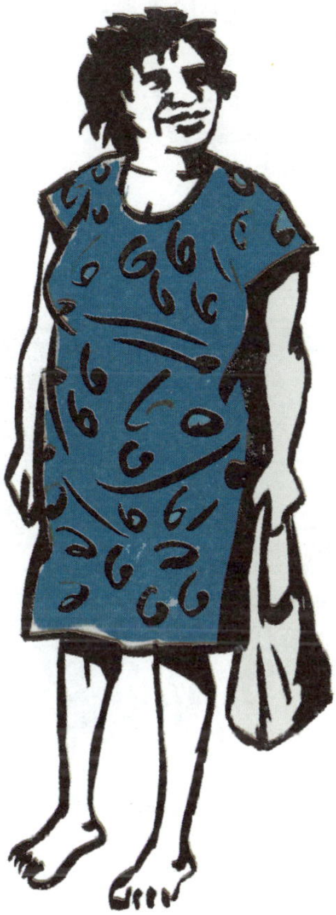

What happened
to Roxanne

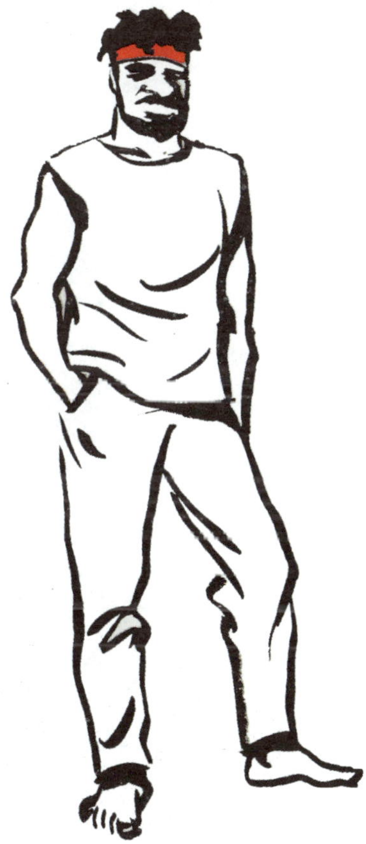

and her brother...

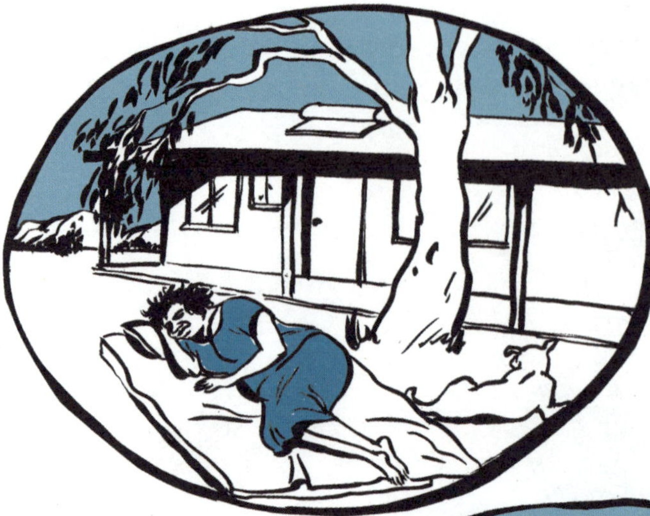

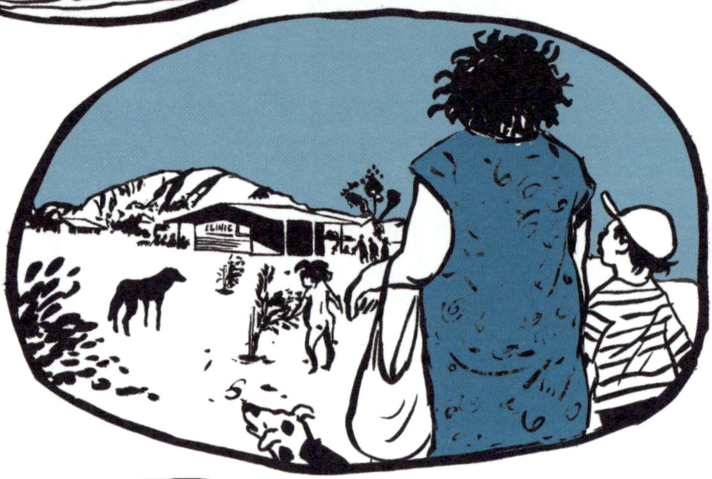
CLINIC

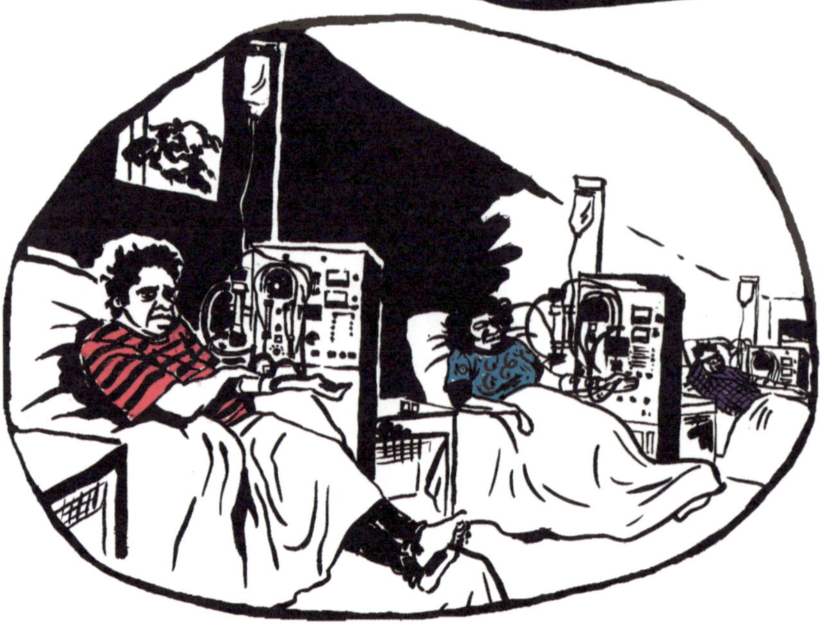

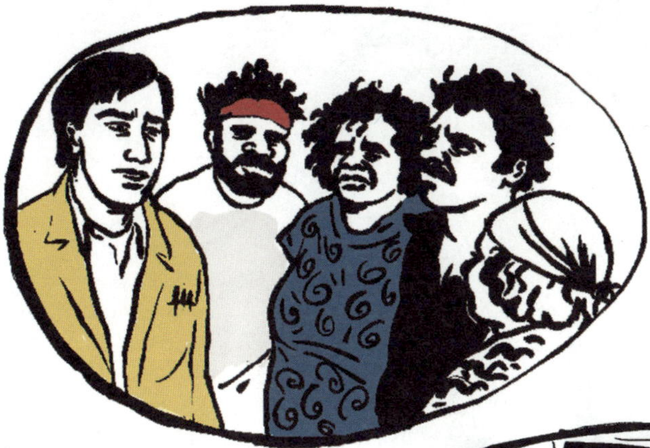

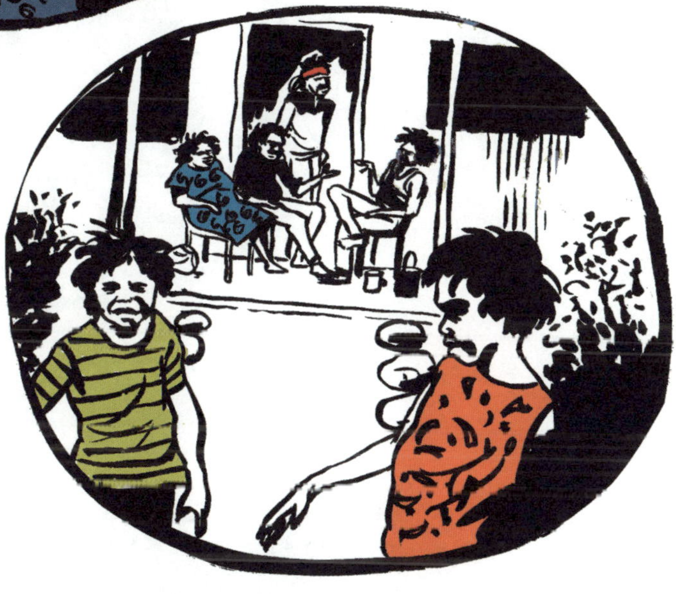

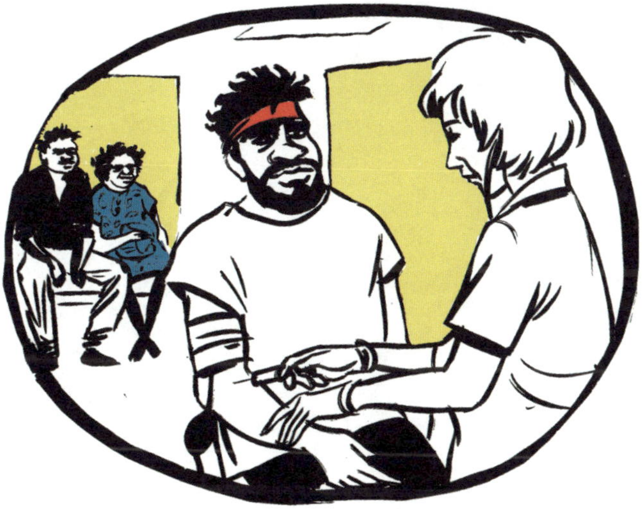

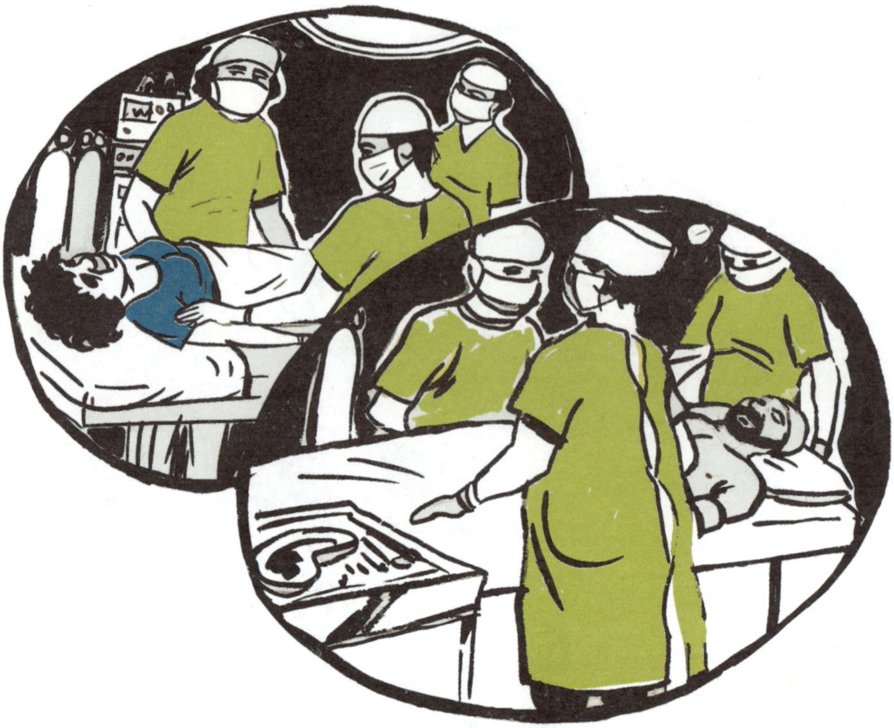

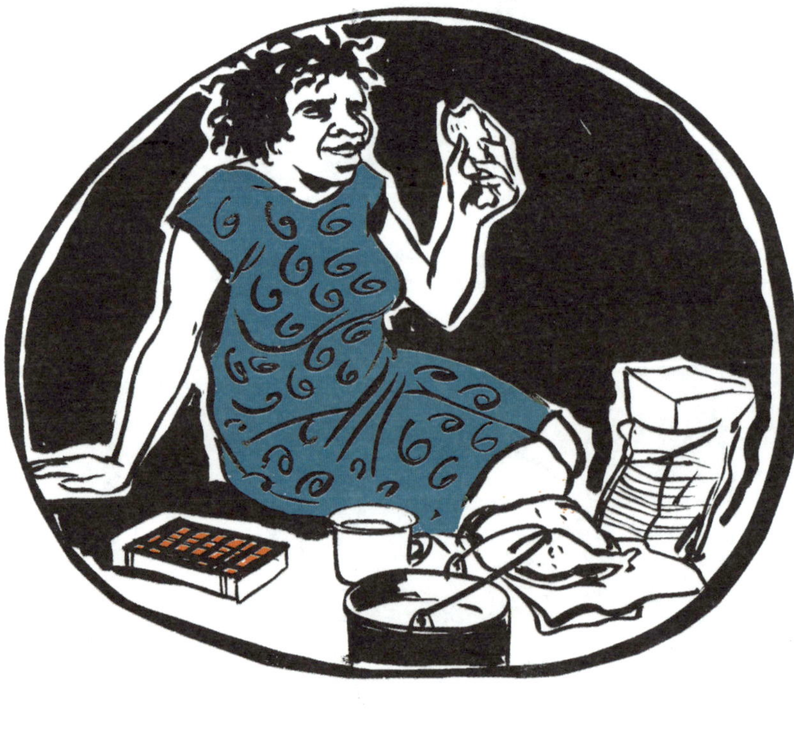

But

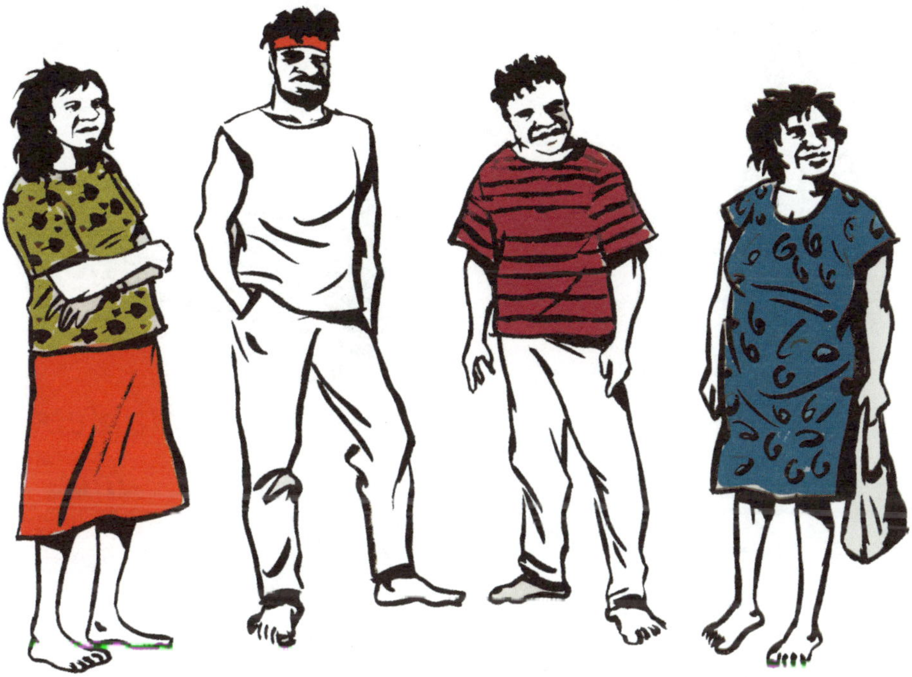

Vera, Roxanne's brother, Maxie and Roxanne have to look after themselves well. They must be careful all the time.

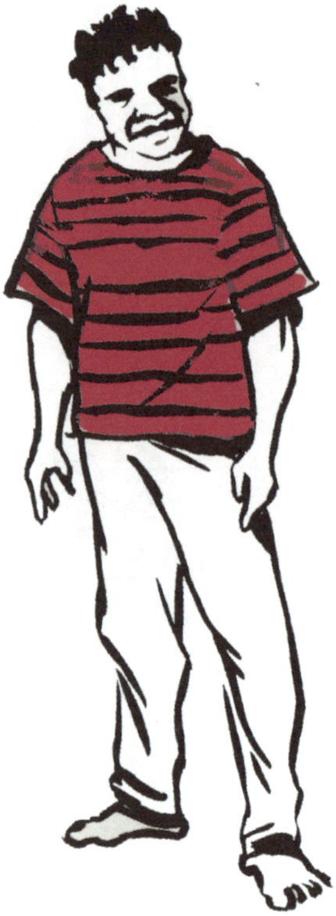

Maxie has a transplant (another kidney) so he

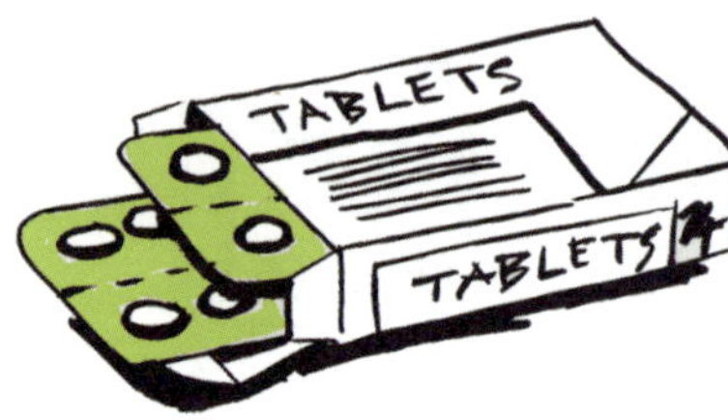

must take special tablets **every single day** — and never miss

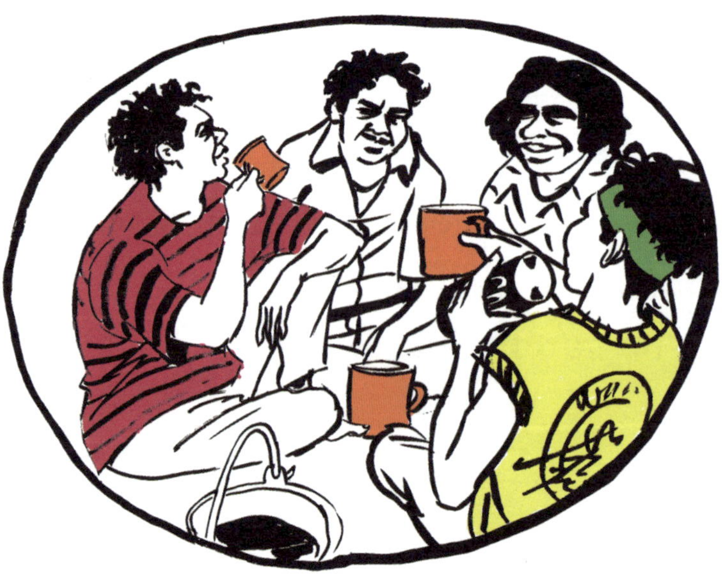

and look after himself.

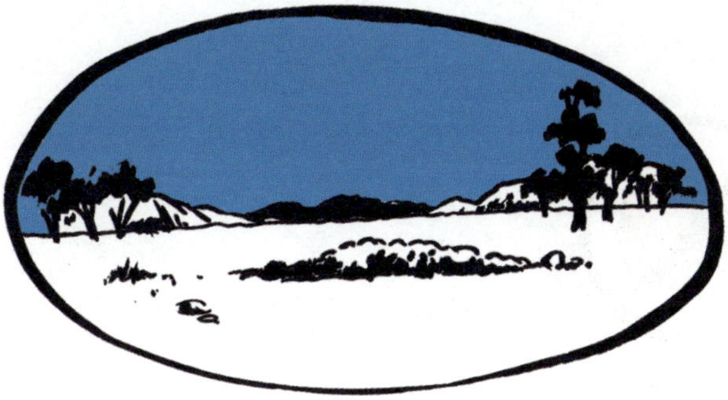

Archie was on the machine
He **should** have...

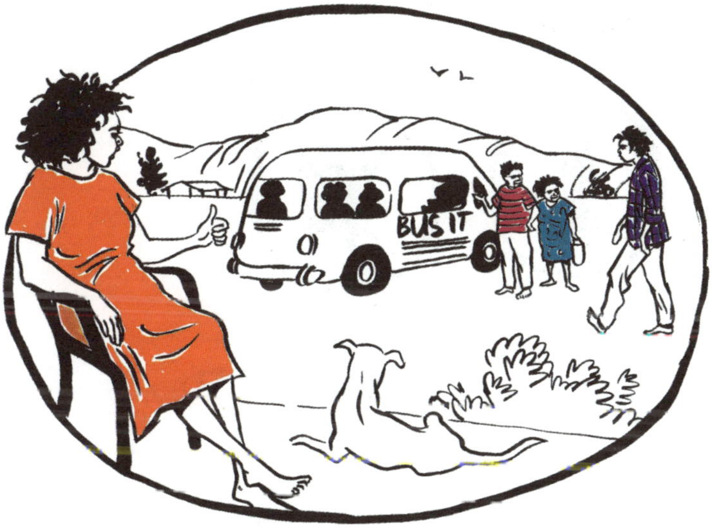

...gone to the machine every time,
and not missed out...

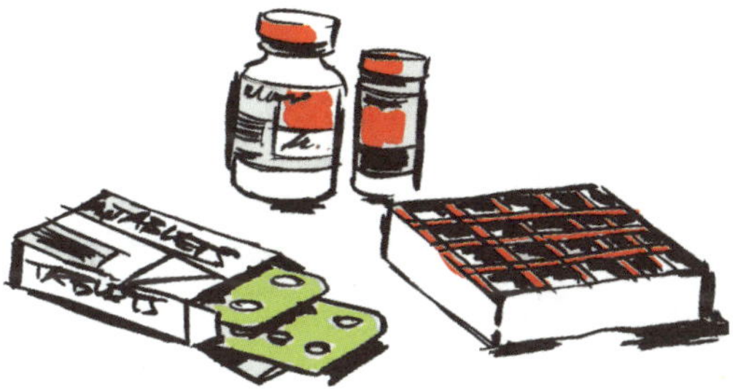

...taken his tablets
every day...

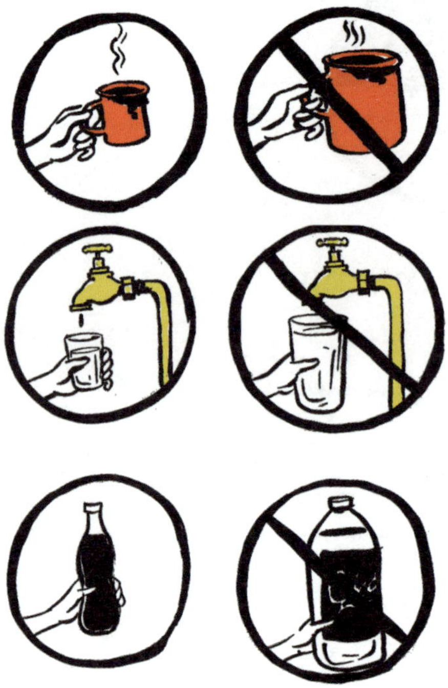

...drunk only a little bit each day...

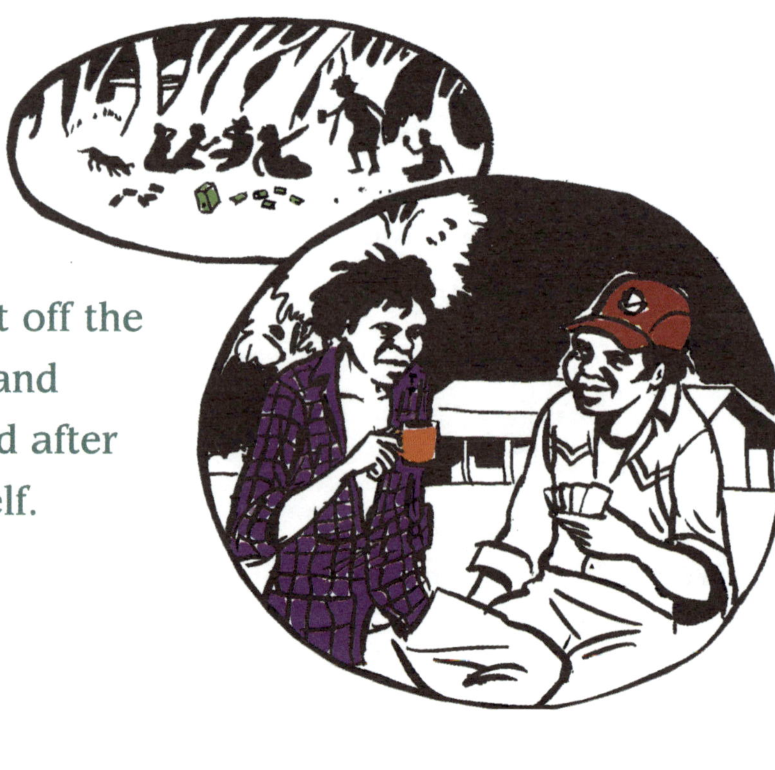

...kept off the grog and looked after himself.

Vera has to

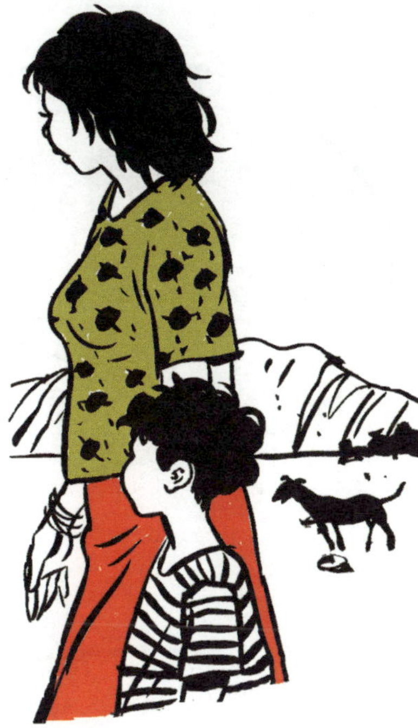

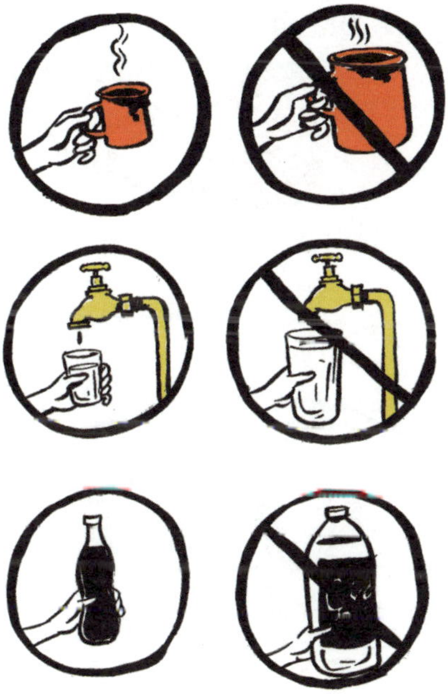

drink only a little
bit each day...

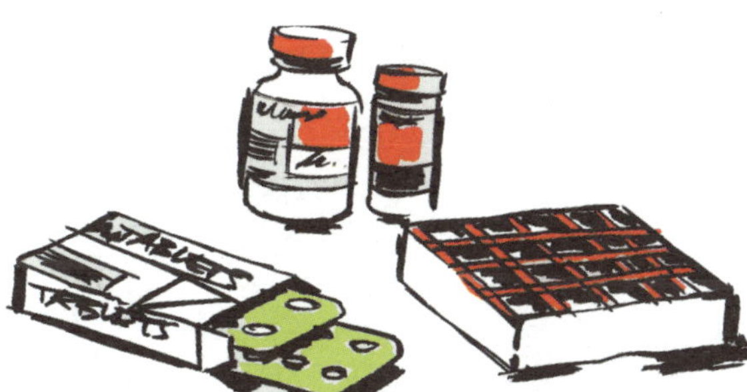

take all her tablets every day...

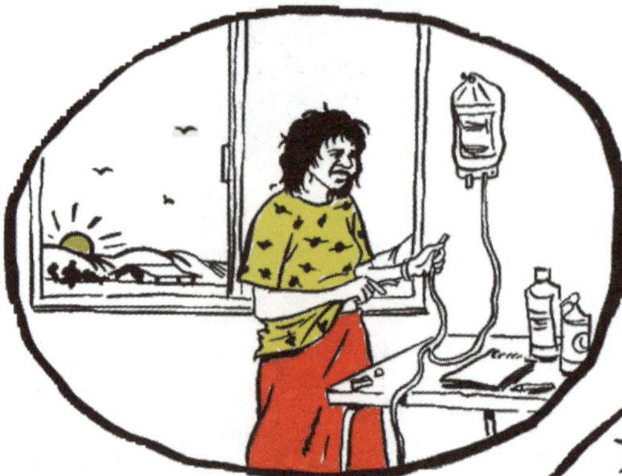

...change the bag 4 times every day...

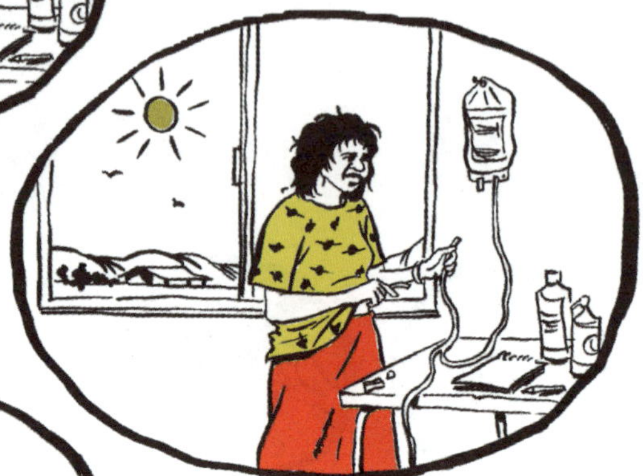

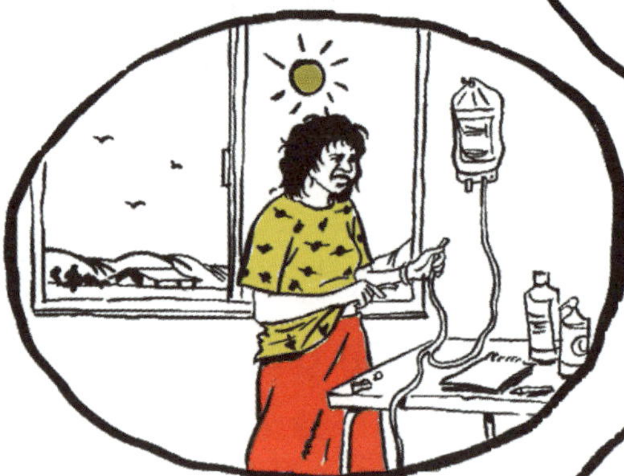

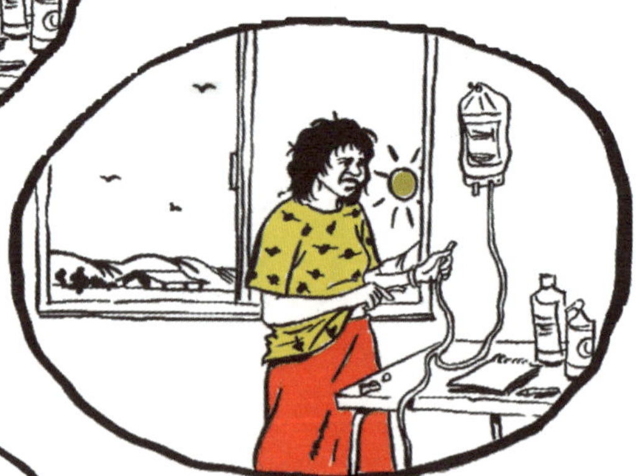

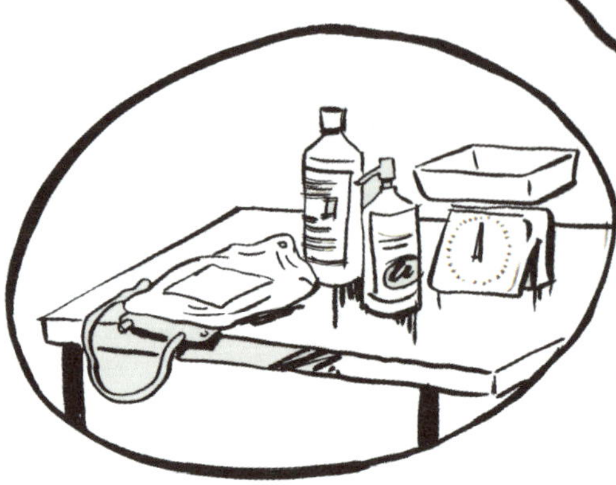

keep her gear clean and tidy.

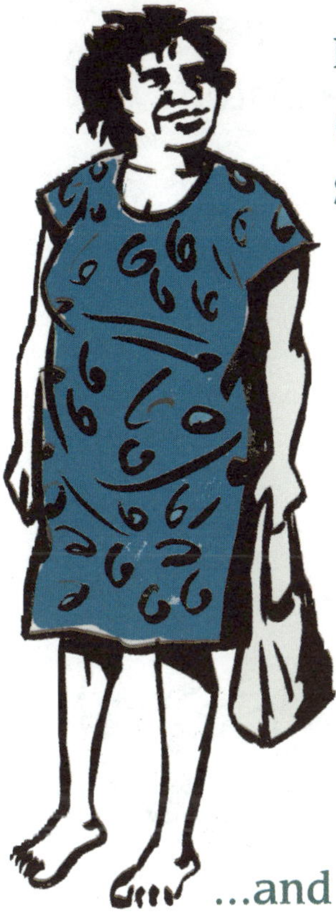

Roxanne has a transplant
(another kidney).
She must...

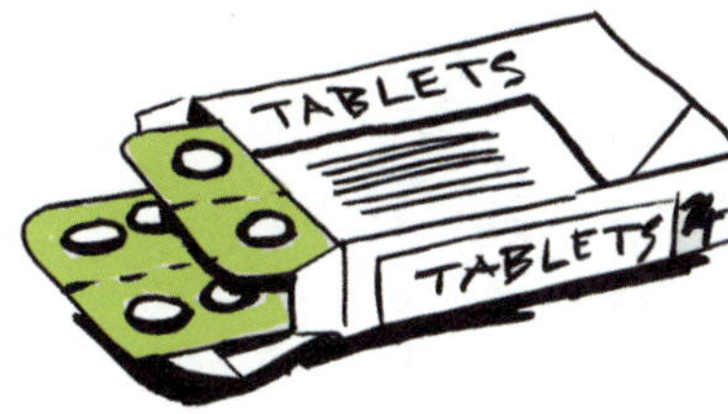

...take special tablets
every single day — and
never miss...

...and look after herself.

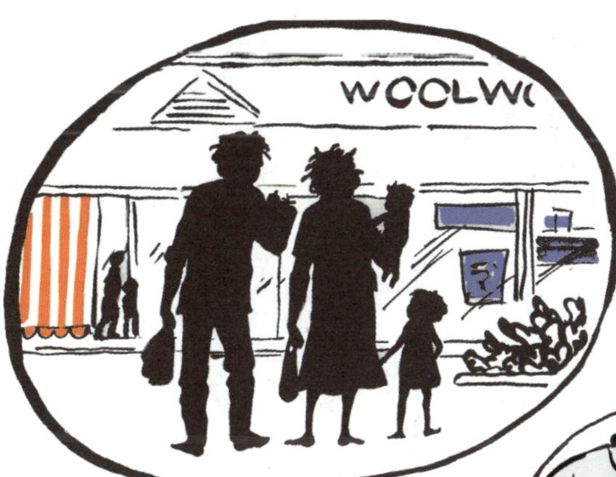

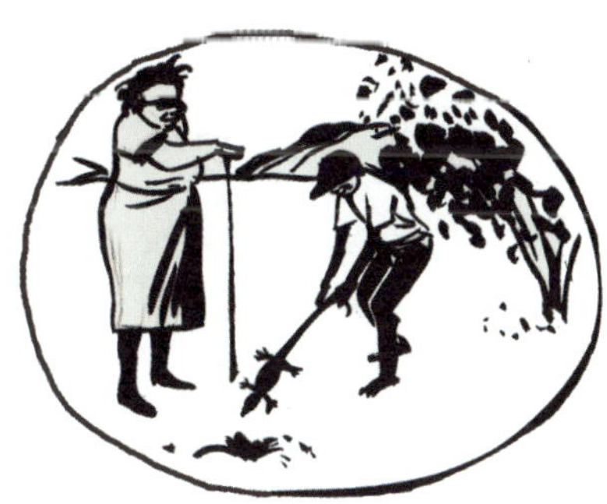

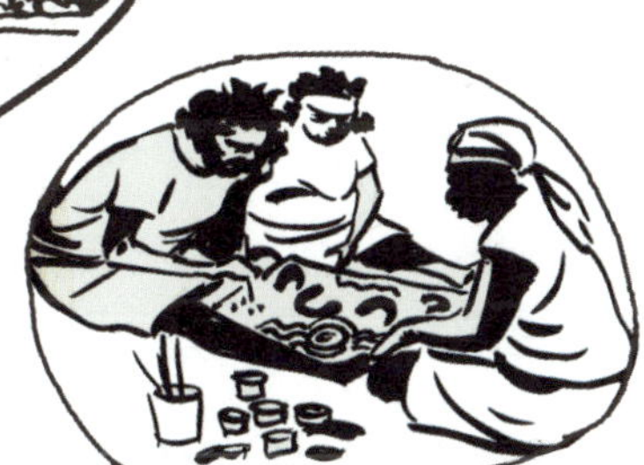

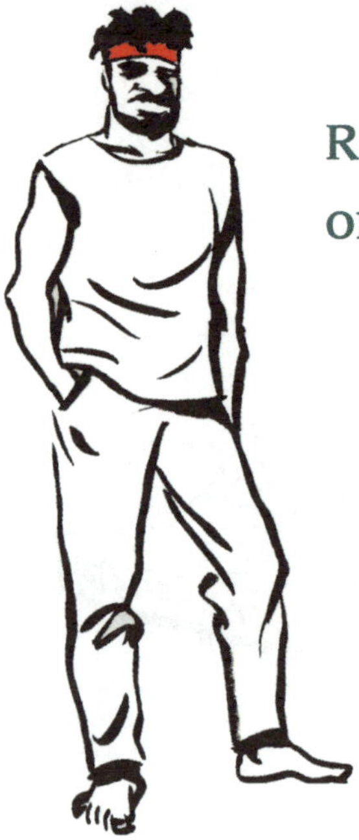

Roxanne's brother gave one kidney to his sister.

He must look after himself...

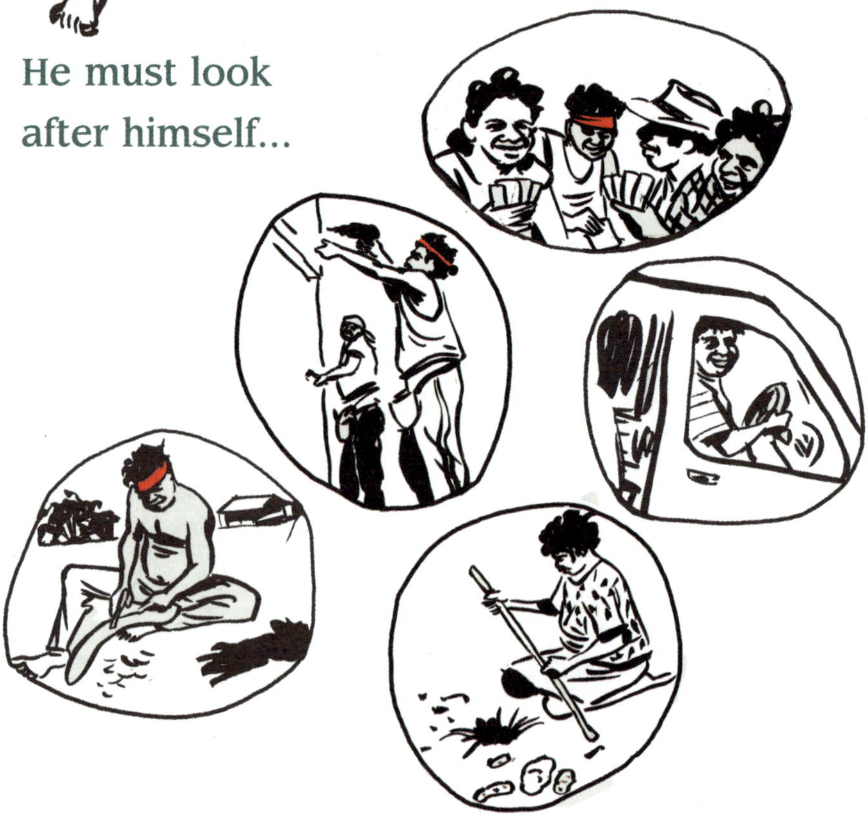

he doesn't want to get kidney disease; he doesn't want to be on the machine like his sister was.